19x 8|14

THE
VITAMIN D
SOLUTION

THE
VITAMIN D
SOLUTION

A 3-Step Strategy to Cure Our
Most Common Health Problem

MICHAEL F. HOLICK, Ph.D., M.D.

Foreword by ANDREW WEIL, M.D.

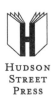

HUDSON
STREET
PRESS

HUDSON STREET PRESS
Published by the Penguin Group
Penguin Group (USA) Inc., 375 Hudson Street, New York, New York 10014, U.S.A. • Penguin Group (Canada), 90 Eglinton Avenue East, Suite 700, Toronto, Ontario, Canada M4P 2Y3 (a division of Pearson Penguin Canada Inc.) • Penguin Books Ltd., 80 Strand, London WC2R 0RL, England • Penguin Ireland, 25 St. Stephen's Green, Dublin 2, Ireland (a division of Penguin Books Ltd.) • Penguin Group (Australia), 250 Camberwell Road, Camberwell, Victoria 3124, Australia (a division of Pearson Australia Group Pty. Ltd.) • Penguin Books India Pvt. Ltd., 11 Community Centre, Panchsheel Park, New Delhi – 110 017, India • Penguin Group (NZ), 67 Apollo Drive, Rosedale, North Shore 0632, New Zealand (a division of Pearson New Zealand Ltd.) • Penguin Books (South Africa) (Pty.) Ltd., 24 Sturdee Avenue, Rosebank, Johannesburg 2196, South Africa

Penguin Books Ltd., Registered Offices: 80 Strand, London WC2R 0RL, England

First published by Hudson Street Press, a member of Penguin Group (USA) Inc.

First Printing, April 2010
10   9   8   7   6   5   4   3   2

REGISTERED TRADEMARK—MARCA REGISTRADA

HUDSON
STREET
PRESS

LIBRARY OF CONGRESS CATALOGING-IN-PUBLICATION DATA

Holick, M. F. (Michael F.)
    The vitamin D solution : a 3-step strategy to cure our most common health problem / Michael F. Holick ; foreword by Andrew Weil.
        p. cm.
    Includes bibliographical references and index.
    ISBN 978-1-59463-067-5 (hardcover : alk. paper)   1. Vitamin D—Health aspects.
2. Vitamin D in human nutrition.   I. Title.
    QP772.V53H65 2010
    612.3'99—dc22
                                                                                        2009053666
Printed in the United States of America

Set in New Caledonia • Designed by Eve L. Kirch

PUBLISHER'S NOTE
Every effort as been made to ensure that the information contained in this book is complete and accurate. However, neither the publisher nor the author is engaged in rendering professional advice or services to the individual reader. The ideas, procedures, and suggestions contained in this book are not intended as a substitute for consulting with your physician. All matters regarding your health require medical supervision. Neither the author nor the publisher shall be liable or responsible for any loss or damage allegedly arising from any information or suggestion in this book.

While the author has made every effort to provide accurate telephone numbers and Internet addresses at the time of publication, neither the publisher nor the author assumes any responsibility for errors, or for changes that occur after publication. Further, publisher does not have any control over and does not assume any responsibility for author or third-party websites or their content.

This book is printed on acid-free paper. [∞]

To my best friend and loving wife, Sally Ann, whose dedication to our family and unwavering support of all of my activities have been instrumental in my ability to communicate to the world the insidious health consequences of the vitamin D–deficiency pandemic.

CONTENTS

Part II
Three Steps to Rebuilding Your Vitamin D Levels

ACKNOWLEDGMENTS

This book has been in its making for nearly thirty years. Without the involvement of my family members, friends, and colleagues, you would not be reading this; it does take a village to put a good book together. I am eternally grateful to my wife, Sally, and our children, Michael Todd and Emily Ann, who not only participated in some of the research that I present in this book, but have also been gracious champions of my career and dedication to vitamin D research.

When Bonnie Solow first called me to ask about doing a book, I knew it was finally time to share the knowledge that I and my colleagues had been collecting through years of steadfast research with the world, much of which was going unnoticed by the general public but could be used to enhance the health of millions. Thank you, Bonnie, for paving the way for this book to finally reach those millions; your leadership, guidance, and enthusiastic support of this project have been invaluable. You are a delight to work with, for your attention to details, good humor, and commitment to overseeing every step in the project's process are a bonus that few authors experience with their agents.

I am most grateful to Kristin Loberg, my ghost writer, who listened to my many scientific presentations as well as stories about my experiences with vitamin D improving the health of Komodo dragons, iguanas, polar bears, and a baby gorilla, just to mention a few. She skillfully helped me weave what I hope is a compelling and convincing message about the vitamin D–deficiency pandemic, its serious health consequences, and how, in three simple steps, you can improve your vitamin D status for good health.

I will forever be indebted to the numerous technicians, students, fellows, and colleagues with whom I have collaborated over the years in the field of vitamin D photobiology, physiology, biochemistry, and clinical application. I am most grateful to my mentor and friend for more than thirty years, Dr. John T. Potts Jr., for his wonderful guidance and counsel. I am appreciative for the support from the UV Foundation in funding some of my research on vitamin D and cancer. A big thanks goes out to Jim and Kathy Shepherd, and John Overstreet for your friendship over the past decade. I am particularly appreciative of the assistance, counsel, and inspiration given to me by Dr. John Adams, Mrs. Mary Aldrich, R.N., Dr. Mary Allen, Dr. Andre Araujo, Ms. Carole Baggerly, Ms. Mara Banks, Dr. Howard Bauchner, Dr. Shally Bhasin, Ms. Rachael Biancuzzo, Dr. Douglass Bibuld, Dr. Heike Bischoff-Ferrari, Dr. George Brainard, Dr. John Cannell, Dr. Laura Carbone, Dr. Tai Chen, Dr. Farhad Chimeh, Dr. Thomas Clemens, Dr. Robert Cousins, Dr. Bess Dawson-Hughes, Mrs. Sheila DeCastro, R.N., Dr. Hector DeLuca, Dr. Emily Demetriou, Dr. Cermina Durakovik, Dr. Christina Economos, Dr. Frank Farraye, Dr. Gary Ferguson, Drs. Cedric and Frank Garland, Dr. William Gehrmann, Dr. Catherine Gordon, Dr. Edward Gorhan, Dr. William Grant, Dr. Susan Greenspan, Dr. Robert Heaney, Dr. Brett Holmquist, Mr. Daniel Jamieson, Dr. David Kenney, Dr. Douglas Kiel, Mrs. Ellen Klein, Dr. Albert Kligman, Dr. Loren Kline, Dr. Polyxeni Koutkia, Dr. Rolfdieter Krause, Dr. Joyce Lee, Dr. Linda Linday, Mr. Zhiren Liu, Dr. Cliford Lo, Dr. Alan Malabanan, Dr. Trond Marksted, Mr. Jeffrey Mathieu, Dr. Lois Matsuoko, Dr. Carlos Mautalen, Ms. Julia McLaughlin, Ms. Janeen McNeil, R.N., Ms. Anne Merewood, Dr. Johan Moan, Dr. Carolyn Moore, Dr. Haraikarn Nimitphong, Dr. James O'Keefe, Dr. Jack Omdahl, Dr. John Parrish, Dr. Ralf Paus, Dr. Alberto Perez, Mr. Kelly Persons, Dr. John Pettifor, Dr. Sara Pietras, Dr. Pornpoj Pramyothin, Dr. Kumaravel Rajakumar, Dr. Rahul Ray, Mrs. Swapna Ray, Dr. Jorg Reichrath, Dr. Richard Reitz, Dr. Clifford Rosen, Dr. Irv Rosenberg, Dr. William Rosenberg, Dr. Josh Safer, Dr. Wael Salameh, Dr. Edward Sauter, Dr. Nevin Schrimshaw, Dr.

Gary Schwartz, Mr. Jim Shepherd, Dr. Leonid Shinchuk, Dr. Andrzej Slominski, Elizabeth Southworth, Ms. Catherine St. Clair, Dr. Mark St. Lezin, Dr. Tatsuo Suda, Dr. Susan Sullivan, Dr. Vin Tangpricha, Mr. Andrew Tannenbaum, Dr. Xiao Tian, Dr. Duane Ulrey, Mr. Demetrius Vorgias, Dr. Ann Webb, Mr. Lyman Whitlatch, Mr. Frederic Wolff, Mr. Jörg Wolff, Dr Jacobo Wortsman, Dr. Azzie Young, Dr. Vernon Young, Dr. Michael Young, and Dr. Susie Zanello.

Thank you to the members of the Boston University Medical Center community, including its executive administrators, clinical research support staff, the nurses in the general clinical research unit, and my tireless assistant, Lorrie Butler. Thank you, Dr. Weil, for penning my Foreword and being such a passionate advocate of my work through the years.

To the team at Hudson Street Press and Penguin, who endured all of my last-minute requests and changes, and whose insights have helped produce the best book possible for you, the general reader, especially Caroline Sutton, Meghan Stevenson, Elizabeth Keenan, and Alexandra Ramstrum.

And finally, my special thanks go to all the organisms of the world who rely on vitamin D to sustain their life, and who've taught me a great deal about this hormone that humans are now beginning to understand, and appreciate, like never before.

FOREWORD

Dr. Andrew Weil

The Vitamin D Solution sets a new standard in health and wellness that I believe will change the face of medicine as we know it. This indispensable guide helps you understand why vitamin D is so critical to your overall health, and shows how you can harness its rewards through a three-part prescription that anyone can follow. Since identifying the body's active form of vitamin D some thirty years ago, my friend and colleague Dr. Michael F. Holick has stood at the forefront of vitamin D research, pioneering groundbreaking studies that have linked a wide array of disorders that afflict up to 200 million Americans with a single common risk factor—vitamin D deficiency. It's the most common medical condition in the world with sometimes devastating, even fatal, consequences. Whether you live in a northern region like New England, or near me in the sunny southwest where the sun shines most days, you could be suffering from a silent vitamin D deficiency that undermines all of your efforts to achieve optimal health.

Contrary to popular wisdom, vitamin D isn't just about bone health, and it stands uniquely apart from all other vitamins. Vitamin D is actually a hormone that plays a central role in metabolism and also in muscle, cardiac, immune, and neurological functions, as well as in the regulation of inflammation. Increasing the amount of vitamin D in the body can prevent or help treat a remarkable number of ailments, from obesity to arthritis, from high blood pressure to back pain, from diabetes to muscle cramps, from upper respiratory tract infections to infectious diseases, and from fibromyalgia to cancers of the breast, colon, pancreas, prostate, and ovaries. It can safeguard pregnancy, support ideal weight management, reduce abnormal cell growth, and stave off infections and chronic diseases. Who would not want these benefits?

The message of *The Vitamin D Solution* is simple yet profound: just as we require a little fat and salt for survival, we need the sun in moderation, too—for sun exposure is our best source of vitamin D. It's a well-documented fact that sunlight is necessary for human survival, but we've been brainwashed into thinking that any exposure to sunlight is bad. This is both unfortunate and untrue. There is really no substantiated scientific evidence to suggest that moderate sun exposure significantly increases risks of benign cancers or, and more importantly, the most deadly form of skin cancer, melanoma. Dr. Holick shows you how to safely and sensibly take advantage of sunlight during certain times of the day and year to build and maintain your natural levels of vitamin D without increasing your risk for skin cancer. As part of his three-part strategy, he also explains the role and importance of calcium in combination with vitamin D, and tells you how much you need in the form of supplements to optimize your health.

Throughout this book, Dr. Holick shares fascinating case studies that have defined and shaped his work over the past thirty years, some of which reveal the devastating consequences of vitamin D deficiency even in a country like the United States, where health care is considered to be so advanced. I have great respect for him as a clinician, researcher, and educator.

We are lucky to be living during an exciting transformation of medicine and health care. We have more knowledge about health than ever before, yet we continue to suffer from serious diseases that are largely preventable through simple lifestyle changes. I have devoted the past thirty years to developing, practicing, and teaching others about the principles of integrative medicine, which emphasizes prevention through attention to lifestyle. In 1994, I established the Program in Integrative Medicine, now the Arizona Center for Integrative Medicine, a Center of Excellence of the University of Arizona College of Medicine. Its main work is the education of physicians, nurse practitioners, medical students and residents, and other health care providers, and one of its initiatives is to create a robust field of nutritional medicine. Our curriculum includes the same valuable lessons and strategies that Dr. Holick has developed through his life's work.

The Vitamin D Solution is a very practical guide for maintaining optimum health. Just as Dr. Holick prescribes, I take a daily vitamin D supplement and also get some unprotected, regular, sensible sun exposure while swimming in my pool. Once you have read this book, I am sure you will want to do the same.

INTRODUCTION

From NASA to the National Zoo

By the time we reach adulthood, most of us have developed a general sense of what's good and bad for our health. Eating fresh fruits and vegetables: good. Drinking a bottle of whiskey a day: bad. Exercising a few days a week: good. Basking in the sun without sunscreen: bad.

I agree with the first three ideas but emphatically disagree with the notion that sunbathing is always bad. And I'm going to prove it to you in this book. In fact, I'm going to show you—backed by more than thirty years of science, including some astonishing discoveries in just the last few years alone—how valuable and necessary the sun is in powering up your health, enhancing your well-being, staving off typical causes of disease, and extending your life.

If I had to give you a single secret ingredient that could apply to the prevention—and treatment, in many cases—of heart disease, common cancers, stroke, infectious diseases from influenza to tuberculosis, type 1 and 2 diabetes, dementia, depression, insomnia, muscle weakness, joint pain, fibromyalgia, osteoarthritis, rheumatoid arthritis, osteoporosis, psoriasis, multiple sclerosis, and hypertension, it would be this: vitamin D.

Surprised? I actually like to start with the fact that we suffer from a serious shortfall in this vitamin that threatens our livelihood and longevity. I have been traveling around the world not only lecturing about vitamin D but also hearing from physicians how common vitamin D deficiency is. It's not only the most common nutritional deficiency in the world, but it's also the most common medical condition, affecting at least one billion people.

- 50 percent to 100 percent of children living in Europe and the United States are at high risk of being vitamin D deficient.

- A recent study revealed that there's been a 22 percent reduction in vitamin D levels in the general U.S. population in the past decade.

- In 2009 researchers from Harvard and the University of Colorado revealed that 70 percent of whites, 90 percent of Hispanics, and 97 percent of blacks in the United States have insufficient blood levels of vitamin D; their study was published in the *Archives of Internal Medicine*.

- Near the equator—in South Africa, Saudi Arabia, India, Australia, Brazil, or Mexico, for example—it's been estimated that between 30 percent and upwards of 80 percent of children and adults who have minimum sun exposure are vitamin D deficient or insufficient.

Three out of every four Americans are deficient in vitamin D, up from one out of two twenty years ago.

You may wonder: Why is this happening and what can we do about it? How can a single vitamin be associated with so many conditions?

That's exactly why I wrote this book. One of my goals is to convey to you just how critical this vitamin (actually a hormone) is in our lives and inspire you to spring to action and welcome the rewards that a healthy vitamin D status has to offer. The list of health conditions associated with a deficiency is overwhelming (I listed just a choice few above), and the amount of research that has emerged lately on this vitamin of vitality begs for a book that shares this latest knowledge in a way anyone can understand and use to become a healthier, happier individual. Contrary to popular wisdom, vitamin D isn't just about strong bones and teeth. And you can't get enough from foods and multivitamins alone.

Your overall well-being depends in part on developing an appropriate relationship with the sun. However, it can be a challenge to get the kind of information you need to establish such a relationship. I will provide you with a comprehensive understanding of the issues at hand. Equipped with this knowledge, you will be able to make your own decision about what your relationship to the sun should be. You, too, can learn to use sunlight for health. (And don't panic: if the sun truly isn't for you, there will be alternatives suggested in this book to meet your personal preferences and choices—and satisfy your vitamin D requirement.)

I know that I may have an uphill battle to climb for some readers, who, upon the mere thought of sensible sunbathing, immediately think about wrinkles, premature aging, skin cancers such as melanoma, and so forth, but I trust you'll be amazed by the lessons learned in this book. You may also come to this thinking, *I get plenty of vitamin D because I drink a lot of milk, am exposed to casual sunlight during the day just walking around, and take a multivitamin and a calcium supplement with added D.* Unfortunately, you are still likely to be woefully deficient. You'll soon understand why and learn what to do about it.

A Lifelong Fascination

I've been interested in the importance of vitamin D to human health for more than three decades. When I was a graduate student working on my Ph.D. and M.D. at the University of Wisconsin back in the early 1970s, we didn't realize that vitamin D had to be activated in the liver and kidneys before it was available for use in the body. While studying under young, up-and-coming professor Dr. Hector DeLuca, I was responsible for isolating and identifying the major circulating form of vitamin D in humans as well as the active form produced by the kidneys. These discoveries allowed doctors to prescribe tiny amounts of this active hormone substance to people whose bodies could not make their own active vitamin D due to kidney failure and who suffered severe bone problems as a result. When I was in medical school, my roommate and I made the active form of vitamin D chemically in a test tube and gave it to patients who were wheelchair bound because they had kidney disease and associated bone disease. Those patients began walking again. That was my introduction to the practical application of vitamin D research, and I have worked in this area ever since.

Call it being at the right place at the right time, but from those early years I was transfixed by my studies of vitamin D—captivated by the fact that we depend on sunlight for vitamin D. I wanted to know: How do our bodies make it? What affects this process? What factors regulate it? How do sunscreens and skin pigment influence this process? Can our bodies make vitamin D in the winter? What happens when we live in northern latitudes? How many parts and systems does vitamin D affect in the body? What are the consequences of too little vitamin D? Even after all these years and so many discoveries about the health benefits of vitamin D, I still find this field of science fascinating and needing further exploration.

I have made numerous contributions to the field of the biochemistry, physiology, metabolism, and photobiology of vitamin D, not only for human nutrition but for animal nutrition as well. I discovered the mechanism for the synthesis of vitamin D in the skin of humans as well as reptiles, birds, fish, and whales. I've demonstrated the effects of aging, obesity, latitude, seasonal change, sunscreen use, skin pigmentation, and clothing on this vital skin-to-bloodstream process. I've established global recommendations advising sunlight exposure as an integral source of vitamin D and continue to call for new standards in the government's recommendation for daily vitamin D intake. I've helped increase awareness in the pediatric and general medical communities regarding the vitamin D deficiency pandemic and its role not only in causing metabolic bone disease and osteoporosis in adults but in increasing children's and adults' risk of developing common deadly cancers, heart disease, type 2 diabetes, and autoimmune diseases, including type 1 diabetes, multiple sclerosis, Crohn's disease, and rheumatoid arthritis. I serve on a number of national committees and editorial boards and have organized and/or cochaired several international symposia. I continue to perform studies and have published more than three hundred research papers in peer-reviewed medical journals, including the *New England Journal of Medicine*, the *Lancet*, and *Science*. I've also written more than 200 review articles and numerous book chapters, and I've edited or coedited eleven books in academia. My first book to the trade, *The UV Advantage*, cracked open the door for laypeople to see sunlight and vitamin D from a new perspective. In 2009 I was honored with the Linus Pauling Institute Prize in health research and the DSM Nutrition Award for my contributions.

So Why Vitamin D?

Medicine has long known that there is a clear and undisputed relationship between sun exposure and bone health. Without the vitamin D that humans throughout evolution have depended on almost entirely from the sun, our bones could not obtain the calcium they need to be strong. The childhood bone disease rickets doesn't exist in children who get enough sun exposure and calcium. In fact, one of the most effective ways of treating kids with rickets is to get them into the sunshine.

The relationship between sun exposure and bone health is so incontrovertible that even the antisun lobby increasingly hems and haws about this issue in the face of new findings. When its spokespeople are put on the spot, they usually mumble something along the lines of "Kids gotta drink more milk." In fact, vitamin D–fortified milk was introduced to combat rickets, but much of the milk sold today that is labeled as rich in vitamin D does not actually contain the vitamin D it is supposed to. My own studies have proved this, and that research has been backed by other studies, including one by the Food and Drug Administration (FDA). Even when milk contains the amount stated on the label (100 international units, or IU, per serving), an eight-ounce glass provides only about 5 percent to 10 percent of what the body requires.

Rickets is again on the rise in our society—a shocking development given the medical advances during the past century. But vitamin D deficiency goes much, much further than staving off bone-related diseases in children and adults. Recently, scientists have become interested in the fact that people living in sunny climates have a lower incidence of organ- and cell-related conditions, such as heart disease, type 1 diabetes, multiple sclerosis, and cancers of the breast, colon, ovaries, and prostate. Unlike the connection between sun exposure and bone health, the link between sun exposure and cellular and organ health was more difficult to establish. In part this is because much of what we now know has been learned by putting together research findings from different parts of the world, which was not possible in previous decades. Because it took longer for scientists to make the connection between sun exposure and cellular health, we only recently established what the connection actually is.

And it goes even further. Today there is evidence to link sun exposure and vitamin D to every facet of medicine and health. Adequate levels of vitamin D can improve fertility, safeguard pregnancy, reduce inflammation, help with weight control, protect against infectious diseases like the flu and tuberculosis, prevent strokes and dementia, bolster the immune system, boost memory, and support muscle strength. What all of this really means is that vitamin D may be the most underappreciated and misunderstood antiaging secret. And unlike so many other antiaging "secrets," this one is absolutely free.

No doubt you will be surprised by some of the findings I present, and you may even feel uncomfortable once I dive into the facts about sun exposure and why it's so important to let a little sunshine into your life despite what most of the dermatology community would have you believe. If the noise from the sunphobic dermatology corner has you curious about my scientific rationale for endorsing sensible sun exposure without sunblock, then I encourage you to flip to chapter 8 and first read the truth about skin cancer and the risk of melanoma. Otherwise, begin in chapter 1 and take the journey with me through a comprehensive exploration of vitamin D—a story that begins millions of years before humans walked the earth. I've chosen to save the skin cancer/sun exposure conversation until later in the book; by the time you reach it, you'll be better prepared to take the knowledge in and use it for your own benefit. Though I will say this: studies suggest that those who work indoors have higher rates of the most deadly skin cancer than those who work outside in the sun all day. That's but one fact of many you'll find in these pages that may go against the grain of the established "common sense" that you have obtained from thirty years of the unchallenged message to avoid all direct sun exposure.

I will also present a synthesis of cutting-edge research from around the world, offer a historical perspective going back millions of evolutionary years that will really put all this into meaningful and, I hope, insightful and enlightening perspective, and present a practical— "D-lightful"—plan for rebuilding and maintaining optimal levels of vitamin D. This plan entails three simple steps: (1) using my formula for sensible sun to determine your daily required minimum exposure (with alternative options suggested in lieu of actual sunlight), (2) ensuring adequate calcium intake alongside good dietary sources of vitamin D, and (3) supplementing. Special considerations will be explained for people with certain conditions, such as obesity, pregnancy, lactation, advanced age (older than seventy), epilepsy, malabsorption syndromes, and kidney and liver disease.

I receive tons of questions from my patients, friends, and family, so I've also devoted a full chapter to frequently asked questions—to ensure that no stone goes unturned in settling common confusions and curiosities. For example, does the way you cook fish affect its vitamin D content? Does it matter if the salmon you eat is wild caught or farmed? Do you need to take a supplement even during the summer? What's the best supplement for children who cannot swallow pills? How much vitamin D should pregnant women take? How do you interpret blood levels of active vitamin D? Will I increase my risk of getting a kidney stone? The answers to these questions, and many more, will be covered in chapter 12. Should you have a question not addressed in this book, then post it on my Web site, www.drholicksdsolution.com. I'll answer as many as I can.

Part of the Wild Kingdom

This crusade of mine isn't just about humans. It's about every living vertebrate on the planet that relies on the sun to maintain optimal levels of vitamin D, especially those that are denied adequate exposure to the sun. Take, for example, Kirmani, the first lowland gorilla born at the Franklin Park Zoo in Boston. By the time her caretakers reached out to me for help in 2005, Kirmani was on the brink of death. At just seven months old she showed signs of the bone-softening disease rickets and had severe muscle weakness and risk of seizures, making it difficult for her to suckle and get enough nutrition from her mother's milk. It also seemed to zookeepers that Kirmani's illness had put her parents under serious, visible stress. Her pediatricians advised administering 400 IU of vitamin D (twice the recommended daily intake for human infants), but it didn't do much. I suggested they up the vitamin D dosage to 5,000 IU a day, and lo and behold, Kirmani made a full recovery. She won't grow to be quite as tall and mighty as she should have, because of her brief bout with vitamin D deficiency and resulting rickets, but she survived and is flourishing today. In fact, I was the guest of honor at her first birthday.

This scenario has played out across the country in various zoos where animals are caged and often shaded and protected from sunlight most of the time, and I've enjoyed a degree of renown for improving the health of four-legged residents of planet earth. Twin polar bears at the Denver Zoo have me to thank for their ability to walk after vitamin D supplementation. When the National Zoo's Komodo dragons showed signs of a die-out because the mated pair had nonviable hatchlings, I was called to the rescue. These were the first Komodo dragons in a zoo in the United States, given to the zoo as a gift by the president of Indonesia. After I made sure these large lizards got plenty of vitamin D, suddenly a new generation of Komodo dragons was born, and they are now thriving in many zoos across the United States. (I like to think the polar bears, gorillas, Komodo dragons, and iguanas have been reading the tabloids, some of which have featured my message; when these animals feel weak and loose toothed, they muster the strength to shout, "Call Holick!") But it's not just the tabloids. Other popular publications, such as the *New York Times*, the *Washington Post*, and the *Wall Street Journal* have picked up my insights in the past. I continually field calls on vitamin D deficiency from renowned institutions like NASA and the

National Zoo and advise folks there on how to safely and assuredly rectify a problem. I've even helped develop lighting for reptile enclosures
that replicates natural sunshine, and I advise zoo staffs of how to keep
their vitamin D–dependent animals healthy and fertile. It's a matter of
life and death.

Which means it could be a matter of life and death for you, too.
So turn the page and begin to take charge of your health in a way you
never thought of before. Let go of whatever preconceived notions you
have about the sun and vitamin D, and open your mind up to a shift in
perspective. It can dramatically change your health and your life.

PART I

THE LIGHT OF YOUR LIFE AND THE HEALTH HORMONE

CHAPTER 1

What Is Vitamin D?

Is it a hormone or a vitamin?

Somewhere along the equator a ten-year-old girl is growing up without the luxuries most of us enjoy on a daily basis. She will never learn how to use a computer, order a pizza to be delivered, or drive a car to the mall for clothes and cosmetics. She spends most of her days playing outside near her farming parents, and soon she will join them in tilling the soil. She will never learn to read or write. She will endure periods of poor nutrition and poverty. And she knows nothing about sunblock and probably never will.

Now let's sail north to the United States or Europe, where another ten-year-old girl leads an immensely different life. She is maturing into a savvy user of electronics, passes the majority of her days indoors at a rigorous school, has access to the best nutrition and all the benefits that modern medicine can provide, and will know what *SPF* means long before graduating from high school and pursing higher education.

If both girls continue on their separate paths, the equatorial girl will be at least half as likely to get cancer during her lifetime as her northern counterpart. She also will have an 80 percent reduced risk of developing type 1 diabetes in the first thirty years of her life. In fact, barring any freak accident or untreated medical condition, her longevity overall will be 7 percent *greater.*

The northern girl, on the other hand, faces a host of increased health risks throughout her life, from breast and ovarian cancer to depression, obesity, type 2 diabetes, osteoporosis, arthritis, high blood pressure, heart disease, and stroke. She will be more susceptible to upper-respiratory-tract infections, dental cavities and gum disease, and infectious diseases like the flu and tuberculosis. As a group, she and her girlfriends will break their arms 56 percent more often than their peers did just forty years ago. Because she was born in northern latitudes and has lived there for the first ten years of her life, for the rest of her life she has a 100 percent increased risk of developing multiple sclerosis no matter where she chooses to live in the world after age ten. She would likely lose in a jumping contest with her equatorial sister, who can jump higher and with more force. If she complains of muscle weakness and widespread muscle and joint pain later on in adulthood, her doctor will likely diagnose fibromyalgia or chronic fatigue syndrome when tests don't turn up anything specific. The equatorial girl might never experience such debilitating aches or chronic pain and in fact may develop into a much stronger, leaner, and more fertile woman. If both women become pregnant, the equatorial mom-to-be won't have to worry as much about serious complications like preeclampsia. And she won't have trouble giving birth the old-fashioned way. The northern mom-to-be, however, will have a much higher risk of having an unplanned C-section and of giving birth to a child who will suffer from schizophrenia.

By the time the northern girl reaches midlife and her later years, chances are good that she'll have been treated for an internal cancer (breast, colon, ovarian, pancreatic—take your pick) at some point and been prescribed multiple drugs to combat chronic ailments like hypertension, osteoporosis, arthritis, depression, obesity, type 2 diabetes, dementia, Alzheimer's, and perhaps even insomnia. Because of a significant loss of bone mass, she will be terrified of falling and fracturing a bone, and therefore will have limited some of her favorite outdoor activities, such as tennis, skiing, horseback riding, and golf, significantly cutting back on physical activity. And because she will have lost a considerable amount of muscle strength, her biological age will be much older than she really is. The equatorial woman not only may outlive her northern counterpart, but she'll also be less prone to chronic diseases that afflict her northern counterpart. For this reason, the equatorial woman may, overall, enjoy a higher quality of life—even when advanced age sets in.

What's going on here? The answer lies in the difference between these two girls' exposure to natural sunlight, which is our main source of vitamin D. Obviously, I've taken some liberty in letting a few assumptions go. The equatorial girl's limited access to health care and preventative medicine has its own basket of risks, but let's focus for a moment just on the difference in exposure to sunlight and the conclusions that can be drawn from that single fact. Let's also assume that these girls grow up to exhibit vastly different levels of vitamin D in their systems, which is not a stretch given the documented records of vitamin D deficiency patterns across the globe. If I were to test each of these girls' vitamin D levels, I would not be surprised to find the northern girl's levels terribly low as compared to her equatorial counterpart. And that difference means everything.

The sun is as vital to your health and well-being as food, shelter, water, and oxygen. I'm going to prove it to you through a comprehensive exploration of vitamin D. What does vitamin D have to do with aging and disease?

More than we ever imagined.

Our Most Common Health Challenge

When I tell people that vitamin D deficiency is our most common health challenge globally, the response I get is pretty much the same in wealthy, developed nations: "Well, that can't happen to me or anyone else in my country; besides, we have great health care." And when I remind people that the best way to ensure healthy levels of vitamin D is through sensible sun exposure two to three times a week, a common thread is heard in the response, which is along the lines of, "You can't be serious. The sun is the demon of cancer and aging. No way am I going to consider sunlight as medicine. It's just not possible."

The statistics proving otherwise speak volumes, and you're going to hear about them throughout this book. Increasing numbers of studies are confirming the link between vitamin D and optimal health, and attitudes are beginning to shift. Researchers have long known that the "sunshine vitamin" boosts bone strength by encouraging the body to absorb calcium, but only recently have we begun to see just how far-reaching vitamin D is in maintaining the health of every system and cell in the body's intricate machinery. Vitamin D may be as vital to your heart and brain health, for example, as it is to your bone health. As noted in the introduction, increasing the amount of vitamin D in the body can prevent or help treat a remarkable number of ailments, from high blood pressure to back pain, from diabetes to arthritis, from upper-respiratory-tract infections to infectious diseases, and from fibromyalgia to cancer. It also seems to improve fertility, weight control, and memory.

The evidence is clear: just as we require a little fat and salt for survival, we need the sun in moderation, too. I'll add to that the following fact, which will be fully explored in chapter 8: there is essentially no substantiated scientific evidence to suggest that moderate sun exposure significantly increases risks of benign skin cancers or, and more importantly, the most deadly form of skin cancer, melanoma. In fact, if you were unfortunately to develop melanoma, you would be more likely to survive it if you had adequate sun exposure as a child and young adult. And if you had adequate sun exposure as a child, you would have a 40 percent reduced risk of developing lymphoma as a young adult.

In the past five years alone there has been a breakthrough in our understanding of why sun exposure benefits health in so many ways, something that was not fully comprehended until now. This breakthrough has forced people to take a closer look at the value of sun exposure. I am proud to say that I have been at the forefront of this research.

Groundbreaking new research has linked a wide array of disorders that afflict up to two hundred million Americans to a single common factor—vitamin D deficiency or insufficiency, the most common medical condition in the world with sometimes devastating, if not fatal, consequences.

And the research keeps coming from various labs around the world investigating vitamin D. As I write this, doctors at the University of

Pennsylvania have revealed that vitamin D can prevent or forestall the irreversible decline in respiratory function over time that leaves many asthmatics even more vulnerable when they suffer an asthma attack. At the same time, scientists at the Moores Cancer Center at the University of California at San Diego have raised the possibility that low vitamin D may be *the* root cause of cancer. No doubt we will continue to see remarkable studies emerge, and you'll be reading about some of the more fascinating and profound studies in the upcoming chapters. It's no wonder that this vitamin made *Time* magazine's list of the top ten medical breakthroughs of 2007. So if you can dramatically decrease your risk of illness and age-related disease and live a healthier, happier life— without its costing you a penny—wouldn't you want to do that?

Centuries of Problem Solving

When you put the vitamin D story into the perspective of human history, it begins with the Industrial Revolution. As the revolution began to sweep across northern Europe in the mid-seventeenth century, doctors reported seeing a new disease that afflicted young children with a constellation of physical signs and symptoms, notably deformities of the skeleton, such as bowed legs, misshapen pelvis, enlarged head, prominent knobby projections along the ribs, curvature of the spine, poor teeth, and weak and flabby legs. The disease had devastating consequences. It not only retarded growth and carried serious risk of upper-respiratory-tract infections including tuberculosis and influenza, but it also had far-reaching effects into adulthood and impaired these children's ability to function throughout their lives. Women with a distorted pelvis often had difficulty with childbirth and were at high risk of dying or giving birth to an unhealthy child.

Several theories about the cause of this debilitating disease called rickets surfaced in the early 1900s, including infection, lack of activity, poor nutrition, and an inherited disorder. Although cod liver oil (high in vitamin D) appeared to be effective in preventing the disease, it was principally used on the coastlines of the Scandinavian countries and the United Kingdom and was not widely used elsewhere. The disease continued to plague the industrial centers of the world.

What was happening was that as people began to congregate in Great Britain and northern Europe, they erected cities whose tightly placed buildings closed off to sunlight the alleys where kids were hanging out and living. Compounding the problem was the gathering pollution from coal burning, which thickened the air and blocked the sun's rays. When these kids started to show signs of bone deformities, doctors began to take note.

"Water works wonders, air can do even more, but light works best of all."

In the 1820s, a Polish doctor named Jedrzej Sniadecki observed that children who lived in the city of Warsaw had a much higher prevalence of rickets than youngsters who lived in the Polish countryside. Dr. Sniadecki thought it was probably the lack of sunshine in the cramped confines of Warsaw that was to blame for this widespread condition. He was able to successfully treat the afflicted city kids by taking them into the country-side for sun exposure. But he wasn't taken seriously. It was inconceivable to the scientific community at the time that exposure of skin to sunlight could have any impact on the skeleton. Indeed, it would take another seventy years before the British Medical Association in 1889 reported that rickets was rarely seen in the rural districts of the British Isles but was prevalent in large industrialized towns, suggesting that lack of sun exposure was responsible for the high incidence of rickets.

A year later, a British doctor collected clinical observations from a number of his colleagues throughout the British Empire and the Orient and found that rickets abounded in the industrialized centers of Great Britain, whereas the impoverished cities of China, Japan, and India, where people lived in squalor and had poor nutrition, were spared from this bone-deforming disease. But like Dr. Sniadecki, this early vision-ary's findings weren't taken seriously. Although the exact relationship between sunlight and bone development was not yet understood, a health movement was pioneered by Arnold Rikli at the end of the 1800s with this motto: "Water works wonders, air can do even more, but [sun] light works best of all."

It was difficult for the scientific community to embrace the concept that the simple remedy of exposure to sunlight could cure this bone-deforming disease, and little was done to use these insightful observations for the prevention and cure of rickets. When scientists began investigating the connection between sunlight and health, it was initially believed that the warmth generated by the sun conferred the health benefits. It was Sir Everard Home, who, in the late 1700s and early 1800s, deduced that it wasn't the heat of the sun's radiation but rather the occurrence of a chemical effect on the body caused by the sun that produced sunburn. Home also showed that dark-skinned people had a natural resistance to sunburn.

By 1900, it was estimated that 80 percent of the children living in the industrialized cities of northern Europe and the northeastern United States were afflicted with rickets. Almost one hundred years after Dr. Sniadecki's first report, a German physician by the name of Kurt Huldschinsky reported that exposure to ultraviolet radiation from a mercury arc lamp was an effective method of curing patients with severe rickets. He cleverly demonstrated that the effect of phototherapy was not a direct effect on the skeleton, inasmuch as exposure of one arm had an equal and dramatic effect on the cure of rickets in both arms. People thought he was nuts for irradiating sick kids with a mercury arc lamp (mind you, this was long before skin cancer became part of the conversation), but some took his idea to heart. Two years later, in 1921, two New York doctors (Hess and Unger) exposed eight children suffering from rickets to sunlight on the rooftop of a New York City hospital. They showed through X-ray examination marked improvement in each child. Finally, the scientific community was ready to listen.

In the early 1930s, the U.S. government set up an agency that recommended to parents that they put their children outside for a reasonable amount of sun exposure. Several manufacturers also began to produce ultraviolet (UV) lamps that were then sold in local pharmacies throughout the 1930s, '40s, and '50s. I know, difficult to believe given today's attitude on ultraviolet radiation.

Heliotherapy Takes Hold

By the beginning of the twentieth century, scientists had determined that it was the UV radiation in sunlight that stimulated the production of vitamin D in the human body. They deduced that this was important for a variety of health reasons. Based on findings that the vitamin D created by sun exposure improved bone health, the dairy industries of Europe and the United States started fortifying milk with vitamin D. A craze was under way, and vitamin D fortification was being touted by food and beverage manufacturers ad nauseam. Products as varied as Bond bread, Richter's hot dogs, Twang soda, and even Schlitz beer were sold with the promise of delivering vitamin D.

The first few decades of the twentieth century were the heyday of photobiology and heliotherapy. Photobiology is the branch of science that investigates the effect of natural and artificial radiation on all life forms; heliotherapy focuses on the sun's abilities to heal the sick. Photobiologists and heliotherapists were credited with developing effective treatments for rickets, tuberculosis, and the skin disorder psoriasis. Hospitals all over Europe and the United States built solaria and balconies so they could offer their patients a pleasant place to enjoy the sun's healing rays. In Boston, the then Children's Hospital put rachitic children on a boat and had them exposed to direct sunlight, which they could not get in the crowded, polluted downtown air. This gave rise to the Boston Floating Hospital, which still exists today (as the Floating Hospital for Children) at Tufts Medical Center. In 1903, photobiologist Dr. Niels Ryberg Finsen won the Nobel Prize for medicine after successfully demonstrating that exposure to sunlight cured many diseases, including lupus vulgaris, or tuberculosis of the skin.

Rickets on the Rise

It's hard to imagine a government recommending the deliberate exposure of children to sunlight. But our government did just that in 1931 when it set up an agency to encourage parents to expose their children to sunlight to prevent rickets. But there's been a 180-degree turn in just the last forty years. Today, parents are likely to be accused of child endangerment or abuse if they let their kids roam sunscreen-free in playgrounds and at the beach. This all comes with a serious consequence.

Rickets is not a thing of the past. It's been on the rise lately, and in cities like Boston we see half a dozen cases a year. The main reason this is happening is that human breast milk today hardly contains any vitamin D, and without adequate sun exposure or a vitamin D supplement, infants are at a high risk of developing rickets. In fact, in one of my studies we looked at forty newborn babies whose mothers were seemingly doing everything right before giving birth. Seventy percent of them took prenatal vitamins, 90 percent drank fortified milk, and all ate fish—one of the best dietary sources for vitamin D—regularly during their pregnancy. Upon giving birth, 76 percent of the moms and a full 81 percent of the newborns were vitamin D deficient.

In all, 90 percent to 95 percent of most people's vitamin D requirement comes from casual exposure to sunlight.

Another reason rickets is cropping up again with increasing frequency is that many kids these days spend too much time indoors and out of the sun or are slathered in sunscreen and made to wear protective clothing before they go out to play. Even more alarming is a new epidemic in which bone formation in children appears normal but is actually much softer than it should be. Girls today break their arms 56 percent more often than their peers did forty years ago. Boys break their arms 32 percent more often. Just last year, the American Academy of Pediatrics felt compelled to double its recommended daily vitamin D intake for newborns, children, and adolescents, citing concern over rising levels of rickets as well as the explosion of new evidence demonstrating that higher vitamin D intake may help prevent a wide variety of diseases. Eventually, even the American Academy of Dermatology, which had been having the hardest time accepting recent statistics on rickets and accompanying literature on vitamin D, chimed in.

In July of 2009, the American Academy of Dermatology issued a "revised position statement on vitamin D after an updated review of the increasing body of scientific literature on this vitamin and its importance for optimal health." While still extremely gun-shy about endorsing sensible sun exposure (in fact, the statement plainly reminded members about the dangers of UV radiation in the development of skin cancer, saying, "Vitamin D should not be obtained from unprotected exposure to ultraviolet radiation"), the academy urged its members to remain vigilant about the importance of vitamin D and to pay attention to patients who are at high risk of deficiency. It said that those who are at risk for a deficiency should be encouraged to up their vitamin D intake through diet and supplements—not through sun exposure. I am happy to see this baby-step forward, even though the academy still cannot fathom sensible sun exposure as an option that could be more effective and beneficial overall. I was amused to learn that when dermatologists in Australia had their own vitamin D levels checked, 87 percent of them were deficient! Indeed, the proof is in their own pudding. The doctrine of dermatology will take time to rewrite, but in the meantime, each one of us can establish and follow our own canon of health.

Poor bone health and childhood rickets is just the tip of the vitamin D iceberg. Increasing numbers of adults are developing a vitamin D deficiency–related bone condition known as osteomalacia (pronounced os-tee-oh-muh-LAY-shuh), sometimes called "adult rickets." Unlike the brittle-bone disease osteoporosis, which doesn't cause bone pain and is more common in older adults, osteomalacia is characterized by vague but often intense bone and muscles aches and is frequently misdiagnosed as fibromyalgia, chronic fatigue syndrome, or arthritis. The "fibromyalgia epidemic" that some doctors refer to may actually be a massive increase in vitamin D deficiency–related osteomalacia (see chapter 3 for more on this important subject). I've estimated that 40 percent to 60 percent of patients who have been diagnosed with fibromyalgia or chronic fatigue have a vitamin D deficiency and suffer from osteomalacia. One such patient who eventually found me was pain free after just six months of treatment to raise her blood levels of vitamin D. Her fibromyalgia simply vanished and her bone density improved by more than 25 percent after the first year.

As I chronicled in the comparison of the two fictional ten-year-old girls at the start of this chapter, a vitamin D deficiency sets one up for myriad health risks across the board and throughout one's life. If you are vitamin D deficient in childhood, you are more than twice as likely to develop type 1 diabetes. If you live above 35 degrees north latitude (roughly the latitude of Atlanta and Los Angeles), you are twice as likely to develop multiple sclerosis. Living at higher latitudes also means a higher risk of Crohn's disease, infections, and high blood pressure.

There's evidence to suggest that if you raise your level of vitamin D to a certain amount (and I'll explain exactly what those levels are in chapter 2), you can reduce your risk of colorectal, ovarian, pancreatic, prostate, and breast cancer by as much as 30 percent to 50 percent. You can also reduce your risk of hypertension, stroke, and heart attack by as much as 50 percent. If you're a woman contemplating pregnancy, healthy vitamin D levels can improve fertility, prevent an unplanned C-section, and ensure a healthier baby who will enjoy a healthier life. Women may lower their risk of rheumatoid arthritis by 42 percent, and decrease their risk of multiple sclerosis by more than 40 percent. And with adequate levels of vitamin D you will live longer.

A Hormone, Not a Vitamin

Naturally, we're disposed to think about vitamin D as a vitamin—a substance that we get from our diets, like vitamin C or niacin, and that participates in biological reactions to help the body operate optimally. But despite its name, vitamin D isn't really a vitamin, and as I've said, you can't rely on diet to obtain it; you do, however, make it in your skin. Vitamin D is in a class by itself; its far-reaching effects on the body are aligned with how hormones act to influence metabolic pathways, cellular functions, and the expression of myriad genes. Vitamin D's active metabolic product in the body, in fact, is a molecule called 1,25-dihydroxyvitamin D (let's call it 1,25-vitamin D for simplicity), which is a secosteroid hormone that directly or indirectly targets more than two thousand genes, or about 6 percent of the human genome. (I'll be talking about vitamin D's two different forms—vitamin D_2 and vitamin D_3. For the purposes of the book I'll be discussing vitamin D_2 or vitamin D_3 as vitamin D, and I'll only refer to specific forms of vitamin D where appropriate.)

Generally speaking, vitamins are organic compounds that cannot be made by the body but are necessary for proper functioning. (The term vitamin comes from "vital amine"—a substance that is essential for health but cannot be made by the body.) Obtained through the diet or supplementation, vitamins are vital to growth, development, and metabolic reactions. Hormones, on the other hand, are synthesized in the body from simple precursors and go to distant tissues where they have an intended effect and make multiple metabolic improvements. In the case of the manufacture of vitamin D, which requires the help of an outside source to trigger a sequence of events, the precursor of a cholesterol-like molecule found in the skin cell (7-dehydrocholesterol; provitamin D_3) starts the process by absorbing just the ultraviolet B portion of sunlight to create what's called previtamin D_3. Previtamin D_3 quickly rearranges itself with the help of the body's heat to give birth to vitamin D, which immediately exits the skin cell for the bloodstream. The fact that vitamin D is made in living skin cells explains why it is not possible to wash off vitamin D when you bathe after being exposed to the sun.

Before vitamin D can act as a hormone, however, it must go through two steps of activation—one in your liver and another in your kidneys. I'll be taking you through the details of how vitamin D gets made in your body from sunlight to its active, circulating form in the next chapter. The process is yet another example of how our brilliant bodies operate and self-regulate to ensure optimal health.

If you apply a sunscreen with an SPF of 8 into your skin, it will absorb about 90 percent of UVB radiation and decrease your ability to make vitamin D in your skin by about 90 percent. An SPF of 30 reduces your ability by 99 percent. While it's true that most people don't put sunscreen on properly, people are now using sunscreen with an SPF of 45 or above, so even if you put on half or one third of the recommended amount, you're still getting an SPF of 15 and reducing your ability to make vitamin D in your skin by about 95 percent. Farmers in the Midwest who had a history of nonmelanoma skin cancer were told to always use sun protection, and they did. When we measured their blood levels of vitamin D at the end of the summer, most were deficient.

Most humans obtain from sun exposure their vitamin D requirement between the hours of about 10:00 A.M. and 3:00 P.M. and mainly in the late spring, summer, and early fall. Because vitamin D is fat soluble, it's stored in body fat and released throughout the winter months, allowing you to be vitamin D sufficient throughout the year.

Hormones are more sophisticated, complex molecules than vitamins. They can act in two ways: first, they can simply enter the cell and travel through the sea of cellular cytoplasm until they reach the nucleus—the brain of the cell—and influence its activity; second, they can bind to a receptor on a cell membrane and thereby transmit a signal to the cell, telling it to change what it is doing in any number of ways. Activated vitamin D mainly works by interacting with its receptor within the cell's nucleus.

From Bone Health to Brain Health

Contrary to what was previously believed—that vitamin D receptors were only in bones, intestines, and kidneys—we now know that vitamin D receptors are *everywhere* in the body. There is even proof that vitamin D receptors exist in the brain and that the active form of vitamin D stimulates the production of mood-elevating serotonin. This explains how it may help reduce depression (or just a chronically foul mood). Fat cells, too, have vitamin D receptors, and fat cells can be more metabolically active (burn more calories) if they have more vitamin D. People tend to think that fat cells are like inanimate blobs of lard when in fact they are active participants in the process by which your brain learns that you're full and don't need to take another bite of food. When you've had enough, fat cells secrete a hormone called leptin that allows you to push away from the table. A lack of vitamin D will interfere with this appetite-suppressing hormone whose job it is to regulate your body weight. And we all know what an unchecked appetite can lead to: weight gain and a higher risk of developing type 2 diabetes. Speaking of which, vitamin D deficiency has also been shown to exacerbate type 2 diabetes, impair insulin production in the pancreas, and increase insulin resistance.

The fact that every tissue and cell in your body has a vitamin D receptor raises a question: why would those receptors be there if they weren't meant to have an effect? Many of us in the science community think that vitamin D acts as a sentinel for your health in that it can control cell growth. This means it can affect the instigation of cancer. If a cell begins to lose control of its own growth and is on a path to becoming a malignant cancer cell, activated vitamin D can come to the rescue by either turning on genes to control cell growth or inducing *apoptosis*—a process whereby the cell kills itself. If the tumor takes hold and begins to grow, active vitamin D has one more trick up its sleeve: it prevents blood vessels from forming to supply nutrition that the cancer needs to survive. Once the malignant process begins, unfortunately, cancer cleverly develops systems to become resistant to the beneficial effect of the active form of vitamin D. This is why it is so important to be vitamin D sufficient throughout your life. Just as a gap in your car insurance coverage leaves you vulnerable to costly accidents, a period of time when your body lacks sufficient vitamin D to act on those ubiquitous receptors leaves you vulnerable to disease. In fact, it is known that if you have lung cancer detected in the winter, you are likely to die more quickly than if you had been diagnosed in the summer. Could that be a coincidence, or does lung cancer have something to do with vitamin D?

Suffice it to say that in some respected medical circles, sunlight is being described as a "wonder drug." Dr. William Grant, director of the Sunlight, Nutrition and Health Research Center in San Francisco and a highly respected scientist in the field, has suggested that increased sun exposure would result in 185,000 fewer cases of internal cancers (specifically, cancers of the breast, ovaries, colon, prostate, bladder, uterus, esophagus, rectum, and stomach) every year and 30,000 fewer deaths in the United States alone. Other researchers have taken this a step further and looked at the global impact. University of California researchers estimate that 250,000 cases of colon cancer and 350,000 cases of breast cancer could be prevented worldwide by increasing intake of vitamin D.

Sunlight has a similarly dramatic effect on high blood pressure, one of the leading causes of heart attack and stroke. People who spend time in the sun or on a tanning bed experience a blood pressure–lowering effect similar to that of standard medications that have unpleasant side effects. In my studies, backed by those of others, I've found that sunlight has a beneficial effect on heart health on par with the benefits of exercise. Put those two things together—physical fitness and UVB exposure—and you've got a magical alchemy of health benefits.

Benefits of Vitamin D in Brief
Bone health: prevents osteopenia, osteoporosis, osteomalacia, rickets, and fractures
Cellular health: prevents certain cancers, such as prostate, pancreatic, breast, ovarian, and colon; prevents infectious diseases and upper-respiratory-tract infections, asthma, and wheezing disorders
Organ health: prevents heart disease and stroke; prevents type 2 diabetes, periodontitis and tooth loss, and other inflammatory diseases
Muscular health: supports muscle strength
Autoimmune health: prevents multiple sclerosis, type 1 diabetes mellitus, Crohn's disease, and rheumatoid arthritis
Brain health: prevents depression, schizophrenia, Alzheimer's disease, and dementia
Mood-related health: prevents seasonal affective disorder, premenstrual syndrome (PMS, also known as premenstrual tension), and sleeping disorders, elevates the sense of well-being

And then, of course, there's bone health. Sun exposure helps build and maintain bone density and reduces fractures, one of the main causes of death and disability among senior citizens. Humans also need sunlight to control their biological clocks, which regulate mood, and appropriate sun exposure is responsible for keeping down rates of depression associated with seasonal affective disorder (SAD) and premenstrual syndrome (PMS).

Let's not forget that sunlight plain old makes you feel better—not something to be dismissed in the high-stress world in which many of us live. Those who heed warnings to avoid the sun because "sunlight is dangerous" are robbed of the life-sustaining benefits of sun exposure—and the idea that sunlight is dangerous denies basic evolutionary science.

The Complexities of a Modern Epidemic

To say that our fear of sunlight and our excessive use of sunscreen have put a serious damper on our ability to maintain sufficient levels of vitamin D is one thing. But there are other variables that make today's deficiency epidemic a unique challenge. Age, gender, race, geographic location, cultural factors, diet, drugs, and even certain health conditions like obesity, liver disease, intestinal disease, and kidney disease all factor in. People who have undergone bariatric surgery to gain control of their weight have added challenges.

For starters, skin color has a tremendous impact, which is evident in studies done to identify patterns of deficiency. My team did a study in Boston at the end of the summer—a time when you would expect blood levels of vitamin D to be the highest—and found that 40 percent of Hispanics, 34 percent of whites, and a breathtaking 84 percent of African-American adults over the age of fifty were vitamin D deficient. The darker your skin, the harder it is to make vitamin D, because melanin, your skin's pigment that gives it color, acts as a natural sunscreen; African Americans have to spend at least two times (and as much as ten times) longer in the sun to make the same amount of vitamin D as a person of Irish or Scandinavian descent (more on this later).

The vitamin D deficiency in this community may help explain why there's a health disparity between whites and blacks, with a disproportionate number of African Americans suffering from hypertension, heart disease, type 2 diabetes, deadly cancers, and stroke, as compared to Caucasians.

Another study my colleagues and I published showed that 36 percent of healthy white men and women in Boston (medical students and doctors) ages eighteen to twenty-nine were vitamin D deficient at the end of winter. This was despite the fact that they often took a multivitamin, drank at least one glass of fortified milk a day, and ate fish at least once a week. The problem is worse the older you get—42 percent of otherwise healthy Boston-area adults over the age of fifty who participated in the study were found to be vitamin D deficient. The older you are, the harder it becomes to synthesize enough vitamin D. A seventy-year-old has only a quarter of the vitamin D–making capacity that a twenty-year-old has. The good news is that if you expose older people to sunlight a few days a week, they—like anyone else—can maintain adequate levels. But a lot of our elderly are not getting the bare minimum time they require in the sun—sans the sunscreen and floppy hats—to literally get their vitamin D blood running.

That's not to say, though, that youths are likely to have adequate levels of vitamin D. Another study in nine- to eleven-year-old girls in Bangor, Maine, revealed that 48 percent were vitamin D deficient at the end of the winter. Seventeen percent remained vitamin D deficient at the end of the summer. When the Centers for Disease Control and Prevention did a study in the United States at the end of the winter, it found that 48 percent of African American women, in their childbearing years (fifteen to forty-nine years of age) were vitamin D deficient. Dr. Catherine Gordon and her colleagues at Boston's Children's Hospital reported that 52 percent of adolescent Hispanic and African American boys and girls tested were vitamin D deficient throughout the year. The first national assessment of this crucial nutrient in young Americans came out in August of 2009, broadcasting more mind-boggling statistics. About 9 percent of those ages one to twenty-one, or roughly 7.6 million children, adolescents, and young adults, are deficient, while an additional 61 percent (50.8 million) have levels low enough to be considered insufficient.

This was confirmed by another study reporting that 50 percent of children one to five years of age, and 70 percent of children six to eleven years of age, were either vitamin D insufficient or deficient. This was new evidence that low vitamin D levels could be putting our nation's next generation at an increased risk for heart disease and diabetes, two of our biggest health problems worsened by the epidemic of childhood obesity. In fact, it was recently reported that teens who were vitamin D deficient or insufficient had a more–than–200 percent increased risk of high blood pressure and high blood sugar and a 400 percent increased risk of having pre–type 2 diabetes (also known as metabolic syndrome), compared to teens who were vitamin D sufficient.

This theme is played out whether you live in Florida or Alaska. It's pervasive, in fact, in all parts of the world. It's natural to assume that Floridians, for instance, would have no problem keeping their vitamin D levels up. But one study demonstrated that their blood levels defy their geography; vitamin D deficiency among Floridians was still 42 percent.

After performing a study on themselves, doctors in India reported that 90 percent of Indian physicians—whether they lived in Bombay or New Delhi—were deficient. They now have reported that 50 percent to 80 percent of adult Indians are vitamin D deficient. More than 50 percent of children in New Delhi are vitamin D deficient. Even in places like Cape Town, South Africa, and Riyadh, Saudi Arabia, vitamin D deficiency has been shown to be a problem.

If you compare your skin's vitamin D synthetic activity in the summer to what it is in the winter, you'll see an 80 percent to 100 percent reduction in vitamin D synthesis in the winter—even in a place like Florida. If you live farther north than Atlanta, Georgia, you essentially can't make any vitamin D in your skin from about November through March. In the early morning or late afternoon, even at the equator with the sun shining, you're still not making vitamin D, because the zenith angle of the sun is so oblique that most of the UVB photons that make vitamin D are absorbed by the ozone layer.

In later chapters I'll delve more into these as well as other factors that compound this epidemic, but in brief I want to mention one of the more misunderstood features of this problem: the link between vitamin D deficiency and obesity. Because vitamin D is stored in fat cells, you'd think that people with excess fat would have plenty of extra vitamin D on hand to make up any shortage. As it turns out, that thinking is wrong, and a parallel relationship exists between vitamin D deficiency and obesity. The fatter you are, the higher your risk for a deficiency. Why? The vitamin D essentially gets locked inside the fat cells, unavailable for use.

In one of my studies, we exposed obese and nonobese individuals to the same amount of UVB radiation and showed that obese people can only raise their blood levels of vitamin D by about 45 percent compared to a normal-weight person. Obese people (defined as those with a body mass index, or BMI, above 30) often need at least twice as much vitamin D to satisfy their body's needs. With the majority of Americans overweight or obese these days, it's not a stretch to understand why a similar number of people are vitamin D deficient. The two epidemics have worsened in unison.

What's more, obesity and osteomalacia often go hand in hand, tripping a vicious cycle that worsens the obesity, the osteomalacia, and the vitamin D deficiency like a perfect storm. As I described, osteomalacia is characterized by extreme bone and muscle pain and weakness. Being overweight predisposes a person to osteomalacia because the excess fat absorbs and holds on to the vitamin D from the sun and diet so that it cannot be used for properly mineralizing the skeleton or for maintaining cellular health. In addition, obese people are frequently vitamin D deprived because they go outside much less, for practical and self-esteem-related reasons. This only perpetuates the problem. When an obese person has osteomalacia, the bone and muscle pain and weakness make it virtually impossible to participate in any sort of physical activity that might help the individual take control of his or her weight. As a result, the individual remains obese or perhaps gains more weight, which in turn worsens his or her vitamin D status and exacerbates the osteomalacia.

Treating a person's vitamin D deficiency can cure osteomalacia and open the world of exercise up to an obese individual. A study I participated in showed that it was possible to increase obese people's vitamin D levels by exposing them to UVB radiation, in this case from a tanning bed, or giving them more vitamin D in supplement form. These treatments may have benefits other than enabling the patients to exercise. Recall that I explained how being vitamin D deficient interferes with the secretion of an appetite-suppressing hormone called leptin, which signals the brain when a person has consumed enough fat. Building the vitamin D in a person's bloodstream to normal levels will restore that process. Those three elements alone—lessening bone pain, making exercise easier by improving muscle strength, and rebalancing the appetite hormone—can combine to have a dramatic effect on an individual's effort to put an end to the obesity and adopt a healthier life.

Much more research needs to be done, but I think there is enormous potential for UVB exposure from the sun or artificial sources to be used to treat people with obesity.

But I Consume Lots of Fortified Milk, Cereal, and Juice, *and* I Take a Multi!

When people express doubt over the possibility that they are vitamin D deficient because they don't fall under any of the usual high-risk categories, I remind them that it's nearly impossible to meet the requirements through diet and a daily multivitamin. As I'll explain further in chapter 10, the current recommendations are inadequate.

Look at your multivitamin's packaging: I bet it contains 400 IU of vitamin D and indicates that this is "100%" of your recommended dietary allowance (the USDA's current recommendation, which is twice the 200 IU recommended by the Institute of Medicine [IOM] for all children and adults up to fifty years old). This is not even half of what you should be getting. And you can't just double or triple up on your multivitamin. This can be dangerous due to the level of vitamin A you'd be ingesting.

People assume that if you have a well-balanced diet, you're getting all the nutrients you need. There is very little vitamin D from dietary sources. It's principally found in oily fish, mushrooms, or sun-dried mushrooms, and in fortified foods like milk, orange juice, yogurt, some cheeses, and some cereals. But there are only 100 IU in a glass of milk or vitamin D–fortified juice or food per serving. (Trivia: Mushrooms are the only source of natural vitamin D in the produce section. Similar to the way that humans absorb sunlight and convert it to vitamin D, mushrooms contain a plant stool—ergosterol—that converts to vitamin D when exposed to light. An increasing number of mushroom growers around the world are now exposing their product to ultraviolet light that produces even more natural vitamin D.)

What about fish? A serving (3.5 ounces) of wild salmon can impart 600 to 1,000 IU, but few people eat wild salmon most days a week. A serving of cod liver oil can provide 400 IU per serving, but even that's too low, and few people enjoy downing multiple servings of cod liver oil every day. It's simply not a practical way to get your vitamin D, and you can get too much vitamin A (cod liver oil not only contains vitamin D but also vitamin A, similar to a multivitamin).

The sad state of commercial fishing can also lead us astray. A few years ago we compared farmed salmon to salmon caught in the wild. Because wild salmon get vitamin D from the food chain in nature, where there is plenty of vitamin D because phytoplankton and zooplankton photosynthesize it, wild salmon contain high levels of vitamin D. Farmed salmon, on the other hand, are fed pelleted food that has very little basic nutritional value. There is essentially no vitamin D in it. When we compared wild-caught to farmed salmon, we found that farmed salmon had 10 percent to 25 percent of the vitamin D content of wild-caught salmon—not enough to boost levels to an adequate state. (For a list of dietary sources of vitamin D and their approximate content, refer to the chart on page 227.)

To eat a sufficient amount of vitamin D (1,000 to 2,000 IU), you'd have to consume three cans of sardines, drink ten to twenty glasses of fortified milk, gulp down ten to twenty bowls of cereal, snack on fifty to a hundred egg yolks, or eat seven ounces of wild salmon for dinner every night.

Many Problems, One Solution

The inescapable fact is that humans have evolved in such a way as to be dependent on sunshine for life and health. Sunlight is the fuel that enables your body to manufacture vitamin D. When your body is unable to obtain sufficient sunlight, it can't make enough vitamin D on its own. Why does this matter? The short answer is that the benefits of vitamin D to human health are many, varied, and profound. As mentioned in the introduction, it's estimated that anywhere from 30 percent to 80 percent of the U.S. population is vitamin D deficient or insufficient. In my opinion, the percentage of vitamin D–deficient or –insufficient citizens is at least 50 and probably closer to 90 percent.

The notion that we have to protect ourselves from the sun all the time is misguided and unhealthy. This sun phobia explains why so many people are suffering from conditions related to sun deprivation. When the body doesn't have what it needs to optimize cellular functions and sustain life, the inevitable decline that follows often manifests itself in exactly the kinds of illnesses and diseases that we hear and read about (and fear) daily, such as heart disease, cancer, diabetes, arthritis, osteoporosis, and dementia, to name just a few. These ultimately lead to a loss of independence and a lower quality of life.

I've touched upon a lot of issues in this chapter in broad strokes as a swift prelude to the balance of this book, which will take you deeper into the vitamin D story. What I haven't mentioned, however, is that we can trace our relationship to vitamin D back millions of years to a time when humans had yet to make an appearance on the planet. Vitamin D's legacy begins when earth and its inhabitants looked vastly different from how they look today. Casting back to that time period allows us to see why and how we evolved the way we did and admire the ingenious making of not only the human body, but every body that sports a spine.

CHAPTER 2

Fish, Phytoplankton, Dinosaurs, Lizards, and You

The evolution of vitamin D and the science of sunlight

You would think that I was very careful and thoughtful in my consideration of what I wanted to specialize in as I was working toward my Ph.D., but nothing is further from the truth. Most students want to work in the hottest area of scientific investigation because they believe that will make them successful. In the late 1960s, when I was at the University of Wisconsin, the biggest topic bouncing off the walls in laboratories and lecture halls was how the body uses energy and, more specifically, how it generates energy in its power-producing mitochondria. At the time, everybody wanted to study energy metabolism and the generation of ATP—the energy packer driving all physiological processes. It was mainly postdoctoral fellows who were lucky enough to be working with the greatest experts in that particular field. When I tried to nudge my way into the field, I was told to go talk to a young investigator who was working in the vitamin D arena. And so I did, leaving the prospect of becoming an expert on the human battery to others.

I couldn't think of a more boring subject than vitamin D. I knew it prevented rickets in kids, and we didn't see rickets anymore, so what was the big deal? Why should I be interested? Scientists in the lab I joined already had determined that in pigs vitamin D was converted to a molecule called 25-hydroxyvitamin D ("25-vitamin D" for short). When

I came on board, I needed to get a master's degree. My project was to demonstrate that what they had found in pig blood was found in human blood. I started my research but soon realized that there was a contaminant in human blood that was not found in pig blood. So I couldn't simply follow the procedure for pig blood and was instead compelled to find another way to identify 25-vitamin D in humans.

That puzzle forced me to develop a whole new chromatographic separation system, which then permitted me to identify 25-vitamin D. After only three months, I had completed the research I needed to obtain my master's degree. Then it was realized that 25-vitamin D took too long to work on the body, so there was still a big missing piece to the puzzle. It was thought that maybe 25-vitamin D had to undergo a transformation to an "active form." So the race was on for three different laboratories, each hoping to be the first to identify this "active" form of vitamin D. The DeLuca laboratory, where I worked, was one of those labs.

Long story short: for my Ph.D. thesis, which I completed about a year later, I was responsible for the first isolation and identification of the active form of vitamin D, which is technically called 1,25-dihydroxyvitamin D_3 (we'll call it either "activated vitamin D" or 1,25-vitamin D). In this chapter, we'll take a close look at how your body makes and utilizes this activated form, one of the most vital hormones your body needs for survival, from a ray of ultraviolet sunlight. We'll also explore the magnificent connection between vitamin D and calcium and see why all the calcium in the world won't keep your bones strong without the help of vitamin D. But before we get to the human factor, we need to examine the evolutionary factor dating back aeons.

From the Big Bang to a Big Deal

An understanding of why we all need a little sunlight starts with an understanding of how we've evolved as humans, or, more specifically, how we've evolved as land-dwelling creatures with skeletons to maintain. Humans have depended on sunlight to sustain life and health since our ancestors slithered out of the primordial oceans.

Vitamin D has existed on this earth for more than 500 million years, since long before organisms could contemplate growing backbones or appendages or walking upright on two legs. At the world-famous Woods Hole Marine Biological Laboratory near Martha's Vineyard, my team and I grew a phytoplankton that has existed unchanged in our Atlantic ocean for the past 500 million years. We exposed this ancient life form to simulated sunlight and showed that phytoplankton have been harnessing the energy of the sun to make vitamin D for at least that long. Photosynthesis of sugar may have its origins in prokaryotes—primitive life forms that had their DNA swimming in their cellular soup rather than contained within a nucleus, which is the case for eukaryotes (where life forms encapsulated their precious genetic material in an envelope)—some 3.5 billion years ago, but it would take another several billion years of the earth's 4.55 billion–year history for life forms to develop more sophisticated ways of using the sun's energy to evolve and diversify into various creatures.

At some point in the earth's expansive timeline, life forms got bored with the ocean and began to venture onto land. But as life forms left these calcium-rich waters some 350 million years ago, they were confronted with a problem: there was essentially no accessible calcium on land; it was locked up in the soil and ended up in the roots and leaves of plants. Back in the bubbling saline oceans, early life could absorb calcium right into primitive vertebrate skeletons. Or they ate phytoplankton and zooplankton (microscopic animals) rich in vitamin D. Land presented many new challenges, especially once life forms got bigger and had to find a way to satisfy their vitamin D requirement without relying on plants. This was millions of years, by the way, before humans came into the picture. Land-dwelling organisms may have started to roam 350 million years ago, but the evolutionary line leading to us didn't get going until about 7 million years ago in Africa, at which point our apish ancestors finally became distinguished from the ancestors of chimpanzees and gorillas. Even then, it took the first 5 to 7 million years after our appearance on earth to venture out of Africa and evolve into *Homo sapiens* around half a million years ago. Humans as we know them today didn't in fact emerge until about 200,000 years ago. By then, vitamin D had been around for millions of years. We are relatively young. Vitamin D is ancient.

So for reasons we don't fully understand, it was exposure to sunlight on the skin—producing vitamin D—that permitted these animals evolving on terra firma to be able to absorb enough dietary calcium for their vertebrate skeletons. The main job of calcium is to maintain neuromuscular function as well as build bones, and these ancient relatives of ours developed a system of absorbing calcium through diet into their bones. This biochemical transport process required the presence of vitamin D, which was made in the skin when it was exposed to sunlight.

Did Vitamin D Deficiency Wipe Out the Dinosaurs?

It's long been suggested that the dinosaurs were taken out about 65 million years ago by a giant asteroid that hit the earth and disrupted the natural balance between the sun and life just long enough to kill sources of food. But there's another idea I think is equally viable and related to this theory of what happens when you block the sun's rays from fueling earth's life forms. The cataclysmic cloud of smoke and debris that spread across the land and caused a perpetual winter after the asteroid hit prevented the penetration of not just sunlight but specifically the UVB rays that allowed these animals to make vitamin D and maintain their huge vertebrate skeletons.

When the dinosaurs grew deficient in vitamin D, they grew weaker. Females began having trouble producing eggs with enough calcium in the shell to survive both their birth delivery and the environment, and a terminal cycle set in that culminated in these animals' official departure from the planet. (As an aside, the pesticide DDT almost caused the extinction of the condors under a similar reasoning; the exposure to the chemical prevented the condors' eggs from calcifying properly. The eggs broke soon after they were laid, killing the developing baby condors.) I sometimes wonder, did the dinosaurs die of rickets and osteomalacia? What if fortified foods had been around 65 million years ago? Could their extinction have been thwarted or delayed?

Because nocturnal rodents at the time had minimum exposure to sunlight and thus produced little, if any, vitamin D, they adapted by maintaining calcium and bone metabolism without the need for very much vitamin D in their diet. Even today, mole rats in South Africa do not need vitamin D to survive. We may owe our origins to these nocturnal rodents in our long evolutionary line, but we, like so many other animals with large skeletons, ultimately evolved to require the sun's energy to build strong bones and help create biological products that play roles in our metabolism and cellular functioning.

Vitamin D made in the skin lasts twice as long in the blood as vitamin D ingested from the diet.

When you are exposed to sunlight you make not only vitamin D but also several other photoproducts that you cannot obtain from food. We do not know if any of these photoproducts have any unique biological actions that would be of additional benefit for health, but one has to wonder. My team and I continue to search for more clues in this area.

But back to the dinosaurs for a moment. When the movie *Jurassic Park* became a blockbuster, no doubt due to our fascination with these awesome creatures from once upon a time, a peak in reptile sales soon followed. Suddenly, kids were asking their parents to buy them iguanas— modern, small-scale versions of their ancestral dinosaurs. My daughter, who was nine years old when the movie came out, was equally intrigued and begged me for this exotic pet. I said yes under one condition: the iguana wouldn't become a victim of vitamin D deficiency like so many other vertebrates in captivity. Each year, 750,000 young iguanas are imported in the United States and Europe, and many of them show signs of muscle weakness and bone deformities by their first birthday.

Our family's iguana is called Raptor, and he and other reptiles provide dramatic insight into the importance of UVB radiation on bone health. In nature, reptiles continually bathe in the sun to warm their cold-blooded bodies and become vitamin D–photosynthesizing factories. In fact, working with Dr. Gary Ferguson at Texas Christian University, my team and I showed that vitamin D–deficient reptiles spent more time in the sun than their brethren who were given vitamin D in their diet—proof that even a reptile knows what's good for him when he can't get enough vitamin D from diet alone. When in captivity, reptiles have difficulty getting any sun to ensure their bone health because they live in an enclosed environment that's often encased in glass, camping out in large fish tanks ensconced in bedrooms or living rooms. Even if these glass enclosures are moved near a window where the sun is penetrating, the reptiles still can't make vitamin D because the UVB cannot get through the glass. They may get plenty of calcium in their diet, but without the accompanying vitamin D they fail to thrive. I made sure Raptor had a good source of calcium (low-fat cream cheese sandwiched between lettuce leaves) and installed a lamp that emits UVB so he could make plenty of vitamin D.

Young pet reptiles often have rickets, and older ones have osteoporosis so bad that they begin to take on the shape of an old horse with a swayback as fractures in their upper spine collapse their backbone (this is the equivalent of an old, osteoporotic woman with the profile of a camel). As a result, even the most benign of accidents—such as falling off a perch—can lead to bone fractures, especially of the legs and arms. When X-rayed, many captive reptiles are found to have multiple fractures, which often lead to their death. Responsible and educated reptile owners now understand it is essential to install UVB lamps in their pets' enclosures. Doing this effectively prevents the kinds of fractures previously seen in captive reptiles because it results in much stronger, denser bones.

This phenomenon is identical to what human bodies experience when they do not get enough solar UVB exposure—a weakening of the bones that results in unnecessary fractures.

Homo sapiens Harness the Sun for Health

So we know that humans have been using sunlight to make the vitamin D needed to regulate calcium necessary for bone health for longer than we've been called *Homo sapiens*. Our hunter-gatherer forefathers were always exposed to sunlight. Their skin pigment evolved and devolved specifically for the environment in which they lived, in order to produce enough vitamin D and yet protect them from the damaging effects of excessive sun exposure. Early humans lived near the equator, where sunlight is plentiful, and they developed dark, melanin-rich skin that protected them against sunburn but still "let in" enough sunlight to make vitamin D.

As humans started to migrate away from the equator to regions where sunlight is less intense, and where for several months of the year the sun isn't strong enough for the human body to make vitamin D, skin became less pigmented so it would more effectively absorb the sun's rays when they were available. The farther north humans migrated, the fairer their skin became to make use of available sunlight. The Neanderthals, a distinct human population that died out between thirty thousand and forty thousand years ago and is not related to us other than through a common ancestor around three hundred thousand years ago, were prominent throughout Europe and western Asia. The Neanderthals were the first human species to live outside of the temperate zone of the world and colonize areas where obtaining ample vitamin D was a challenge. Neanderthal fossils recovered from El Sidrón in northern Spain and Monti Lessini, Italy, have afforded us the opportunity to analyze their DNA. And in 2007 the results of those analyses became known, changing the story of Neanderthals in paleontological and anthropological circles.

One of the most startling revelations, though not surprising in the grand scheme of the vitamin D story, has been a shift in how we believe Neanderthals looked. Though they are often viewed as embodying the mystique of the caveman—with dark skin, a small brain, bulging and primitive facial features, and a lumbering body mass, we now have a different perspective to include for at least some of these early hominids. What scientists uncovered through a careful examination of their DNA was a mutation in the so-called MC1R gene that codes for a protein involved in the production of the skin pigment melanin. Melanin also protects the skin from UV radiation. This has led scientists to think some of these early human species struggling to survive in northern climates probably had red hair and fair complexions, much like modern-day humans of Celtic origin. In today's humans of European descent, mutations in the MC1R gene are thought to be responsible for red hair and pale skin because the mutation halts the activity of this melanin-producing protein. The mutation seen in Neanderthal genes is not exactly the same as the one documented in modern humans, but the effect appears to be similar.

Interestingly enough, it's also been surmised that Neanderthals suffered from vitamin D deficiency, which may explain the popular hunched-over ape-man image of a Neanderthal. Complexion-wise, they may have been devolving away from their darker-skinned African ancestors so they could absorb more UVB and thus make more vitamin D. Whether their vitamin D deficiency was partly or significantly to blame for their die-out is anyone's guess. Debate still rages as to how this early species of humans left the planet. Many scholars believe the Neanderthals lived during an ice age, which contributed to poor diet and lack of exposure to the sun. Others blame an invading new population of humans better equipped to survive, for one thing is certain: when the Cro-Magnons emerged, the Neanderthals' last days on earth were looming.

Eventually, humans couldn't migrate any farther north because there wasn't enough sun to make the vitamin D needed to survive. Then something fascinating happened—humans developed the means to harvest the seas for vitamin D–rich fish and mammals of the sort still traditionally eaten by Eskimos and Scandinavians, which enable people to live in climates with very little vitamin D–producing sunlight.

Even today, people with fair skin don't require much exposure to sunlight to make enough vitamin D to be healthy, and people with dark skin are naturally well protected against sunburn. Conversely, people with fair skin get sunburned quite easily and may be susceptible to non-melanoma skin cancer, whereas dark-complexioned people more easily become vitamin D deficient when living in northern climates.

From the beginning of recorded time, humans have worshipped the sun for its therapeutic and life-saving properties. This can be seen in cave paintings that show that ancient people believed exposure to sunlight was necessary for life and good health. Medical practitioners reported the benefits of sun exposure on heart health six thousand years ago, in the time of the ancient Egyptian pharaohs, including Akhenaton. In a famous hieroglyphic drawn during this time, Akhenaton, his wife, Nefertiti, and their children are pictured being blessed by the many "hands" of the sun. Sun therapy was also praised by the legendary Hippocrates (creator of the Hippocratic oath) and the doctors of ancient Rome and Arabia. The Egyptians, Mesopotamians, and Greeks all had sun deities, and the influence of the sun in religious belief also appears in Zoroastrianism, Mithraism, Roman religion, Hinduism, and Buddhism and among the Druids of England, the Aztecs of Mexico, the Incas of Peru, and many Native American groups. That ancient peoples instinctively understood that sunshine was good for them is not surprising.

The race to understand sun therapy from a scientific standpoint really got under way more recently, starting in the first few decades of the twentieth century. During this heyday of photobiology and heliotherapy, hospitals throughout Europe and North America built solaria and balconies so they could offer their patients a comfortable place to enjoy the sun's healing radiation for treatment of rickets, tuberculosis, and psoriasis. As I mentioned in the previous chapter, the Nobel Prize for medicine was bestowed on a photobiologist in 1903 for demonstrating the health benefits of sunlight.

But something has happened in the last forty years. For more than two hundred thousand years our species has enjoyed a special relationship with the sun, even when we had no idea exactly why it felt so good or why we needed a little bit of sunshine for optimal health. With the revelation that sunlight also contributed to skin cancer and prematurely aged skin, attitudes changed. Big-money interests got behind the campaign to convince us that all sun is unhealthy, so that people would always wear sunscreens and regularly visit the dermatologist. Thanks to the barrage of information that was—and continues to be—unleashed upon us, we became persuaded of this "fact."

For the past four decades the dermatology community and, more recently, the World Health Organization have recommended that people never be exposed to direct sunlight. That has been a major cause of this worldwide pandemic of vitamin D deficiency. Drug companies can sell fear, but they can't sell you sunlight, so there's no promotion of the sun's health benefits. Since first identifying how vitamin D goes from UVB radiation to an activated hormone in the body, I've watched the lobby for the sun retreat. I've watched the rallying cry for more sunscreen and less exposure (notice how that word "exposure" even has a negative ring to it, as if it relates to germs) grows stronger and stronger. But nothing is more powerful than information. And to that end, let's take a tour of your body's miraculous machinery for making vitamin D. It's a big deal any way you look at it.

The Science of Sunlight: From UV Rays to Activated Vitamin D

As mentioned earlier, I identified the major circulating form of vitamin D (25-vitamin D) and its subsequent active form (1,25-vitamin D, the only form of vitamin D that provides humans with direct health benefits) in my graduate-school days more than thirty years ago. Once it was appreciated that the activation of vitamin D occurred in the kidneys, it instantly became obvious why patients with kidney disease had severe bone disease and had a resistance to vitamin D. After activated vitamin D was identified, we thought there was hope in using the activated form to treat patients with kidney failure and bone disease, and maybe postmenopausal osteoporosis. But we soon discovered that this was just the beginning of the vitamin D story. In 1979, the DeLuca group reported that essentially every tissue in the body appeared to recognize the active form of vitamin D. We and others went on to show that every tissue and cell in the body has a receptor for vitamin D. And we began to understand that maybe vitamin D had other biological actions than simply regulating calcium and bone metabolism.

One of the first insights into vitamin D's power was made by a former postdoc who worked with me in the DeLuca group, Dr. Tatsuo Suda, D.D.S., Ph.D. He showed that if you took leukemic cells that have a vitamin D receptor and incubated them with the active form of vitamin D in the lab, it inhibited their growth and induced differentiation, thus dampening their cancerous activity. That was the first clue to the potent biological action of vitamin D and its potential role in preventing cancer. After that observation, in the early 1980s we showed that the active form of vitamin D could regulate skin growth and be used to treat the skin disorder psoriasis. Psoriasis is a nonmalignant disease of the skin whereby skin cells multiply up to ten times faster than normal, causing unsightly raised red lesions with heavy, white dead skin. I was one of the first scientists to prove the antiproliferation activity of active vitamin D to restore psoriatic skin cells to their normal growth, and this quickly became the first line therapy for psoriasis.

All of a sudden, it became clear that cells that had a vitamin D receptor had a wide variety of genes that were being turned on and off by activated vitamin D. These genes controlled cell growth and induced cells that were malignant to either become normal or die. Thus, vitamin D could effectively control whether or not a cell became cancerous.

Spot Treatment

Until the mid-1990s, it was believed that the kidneys made the body's entire supply of activated vitamin D. The kidneys make this supply from the 25-vitamin D in the bloodstream that is created by the liver from the vitamin D that is made in the skin after sun exposure and, to a lesser extent, from foods that contain vitamin D (see figure 1). The supply of activated vitamin D that the kidneys actually manufacture is very small (about two to four micrograms a day, which amounts to about one hundredth of a grain of salt), and this supply doesn't change no matter how much 25-vitamin D there is in the bloodstream. In other words, you could dramatically increase the 25-vitamin D content in your bloodstream by lying on the beach all summer long, drinking gallons of milk, and eating mackerel at every meal, but your kidneys would still produce the same tiny trickle of activated vitamin D. The main job of this precious little amount of activated vitamin D, it was thought, was to contribute to bone health. As the person who had actually discovered the activated form of vitamin D, I was very closely involved with what was happening in the field of vitamin D research, and like most researchers who eventually hit the proverbial wall, something began to bother me.

Here's what I couldn't figure out. In response to increased exposure to sunlight, cellular and organ health benefits were occurring that appeared to be the work of activated vitamin D. These benefits

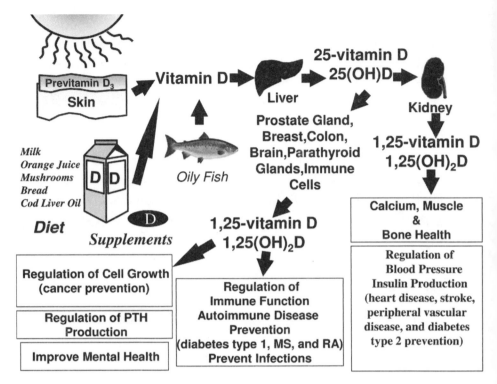

Figure 1. Once vitamin D is manufactured in your skin from the sun's UVB radiation, or obtained from dietary or supplemental sources, your liver creates a vitamin D metabolite called 25-vitamin D (25-hydroxyvitamin D), which then travels to the kidneys to be turned into activated vitamin D (1,25-vitamin D; 1,25 dihydroxyvitamin D). Recent breakthrough discoveries have shown that vitamin D also can be activated within a variety of cells, including those of the immune system, to modulate immune cell activity reducing the development of autoimmune diseases and enhance fighting infectious diseases, prostate, breast, and colon, where it prevents the unhealthy cell proliferation characteristic of cancer.

included lower blood pressure and decreased risk of cancer and auto-immune diseases like multiple sclerosis and type 1 diabetes. However, this couldn't be the work of activated vitamin D if what we believed we knew about the kidneys' production of activated vitamin D was true. There was apparently a connection between sun exposure and cellular and organ health. But our naiveté of how activated vitamin D is produced prevented us from making the claim that one was responsible for the other.

All the while, we were teetering on the verge of a breakthrough in our understanding of the relationship between sunlight and cellular health. Finally, it happened. What my colleagues and I discovered in studies at the Vitamin D, Skin, and Bone Research Laboratory at Boston University Medical Center, in collaboration with Dr. Gary Schwartz and his team at Wake Forest University, was that human prostate cells could activate vitamin D in a way similar to what had been observed in human skin several years earlier by Dr. Daniel Bikle and his team at the University of California at San Francisco. In other words, we were coming to grips with the fact humans have the ability to make activated vitamin D *throughout the body*.

The process is extraordinary. Whereas once we thought that only the kidneys could activate vitamin D, we now understand that a variety of cells have this ability, including those of the breast, prostate, colon, lung, brain, and skin, and probably most other tissues and cells. When the 25-vitamin D reaches and enters these cells, it is converted into activated vitamin D. Unlike the kidneys, however, which make activated vitamin D from 25-vitamin D and send it out through the bloodstream to the intestine and bones, in other cells, such as brain cells, 25-vitamin D is converted into activated vitamin D and used *on the spot* within the cell. After it performs its important functions in the cell, the activated vitamin D extinguishes itself by inducing its own destruction (that way it cannot leave the cell and enter the bloodstream to create an overabundance of active vitamin D, which could be toxic). Because this vitamin D activation process begins and ends within the cell, there is no evidence of increased activated vitamin D in the bloodstream, not even when more activated vitamin D is being made by these cells. This is why scientists had difficulty making a connection among sun exposure, vitamin D, and reduced risk of many chronic and often fatal diseases.

This discovery is significant because we now know for sure that increasing 25-vitamin D levels in our bloodstream via sun exposure, and to a lesser extent via diet or supplementation, will help lower the risk of several diseases—especially those caused by abnormal cell growth, such as cancer. We have also since discovered that the immune system has the ability to make activated vitamin D, meaning that sun exposure may have a role in preventing and treating autoimmune diseases such as multiple sclerosis, rheumatoid arthritis, Crohn's disease, and type 1 diabetes.

My laboratory studies continued to confirm that activated vitamin D is an extremely potent substance that is one of the most effective inhibitors of abnormal cell growth. The discovery by my laboratory and other laboratories that cells throughout the body can activate vitamin D was a major breakthrough in vitamin D research. It is what's behind the emerging realization that—contrary to what we hear so often—the advantages of sun exposure far outweigh the potential negative consequences (much more on this topic in chapter 8).

Add to this the growing body of research showing that sun exposure helps regulate circadian rhythms, thus preventing mood-related conditions such as seasonal affective disorder, premenstrual syndrome, and depression due to decreased melatonin levels. This expansive body of research has had some interesting offshoots, spawning fresh insights into areas of our physiology that we never would have expected. For example, we recently confirmed something that scientists had discovered in the 1980s but that had never been followed up on: It's not just the brain that makes the "feel-good" substance beta endorphin. When exposed to UVB radiation, skin also makes beta endorphins right there on the spot. This may explain why people often feel so good after spending time at the beach or even in a tanning bed.

The Sun's Trigger: UVB, Not UVA or UVC

The vitamin D–making miracle starts, of course, with the sun. Sunlight consists of a mixture of packets (technically called photons) of electromagnetic radiation energy of various wavelengths, from the longest and least energetic, called infrared, through red, orange, yellow, green, blue, indigo and violet, to the shortest and most energetic in wavelength, called ultraviolet radiation.

Ultraviolet, or UV, radiation, consists of UVA, UVB, and UVC. UVC (200 to 280 nanometers) and some of UVB (281 to 289 nanometers) are completely absorbed by the ozone in the atmosphere, so they never reach earth or human skin. UVA (320 to 400 nanometers) and most UVB (290 to 319 nanometers) reach earth's surface to varying degrees but have different effects on your body. As much as one hundred times more UVA radiation reaches the earth's surface than UVB, and though UVA contains much less energy than UVB, it's able to penetrate deeper into the layers of your skin, where it affects the elastic structures, increases free radicals, causes wrinkles, and also influences the immune system and melanocytes, or skin-pigment cells. For this reason, UVA is thought to be a major cause of melanomas. UVB, on the other hand, is the high-energy form of radiation that is absorbed by DNA and proteins and is less penetrating. UVB reddens skin and is a major contributor, over the long term, to nonmelanoma skin cancer. When UVB causes sunburns, it may contribute to melanoma.

UVB is also the only form of UV radiation that starts the reaction in skin that stimulates the production of vitamin D. Until recently, most sunscreens blocked only UVB radiation, which may have precipitated the rise in melanoma in the United States and other Western cultures. That's because sunscreens that block out only the burning UVB radiation enable people to stay out in the sun for unlimited periods of time, during which they are not protected against the deeply penetrating UVA radiation. Without any sunscreen at all, people would not have been able to stay out in the sun long enough to receive the dose of UVA that can increase the risk of melanoma. Thankfully, researchers have now developed "broad spectrum" sunscreens, which protect against most of the UVA and nearly all of the UVB radiation (depending on the SPF).

The level of UV radiation that reaches the earth varies depending on several factors. One of those factors is the stratospheric ozone layer, which absorbs most of the sun's damaging UV radiation. But how much it absorbs depends on what time of year it is and other natural phenomena. As a whole, the ozone layer has thinned due to industrial pollution and now-banned substances previously emitted by refrigerants and certain consumer products such as hairspray. Seven chief factors affect how much UV radiation actually reaches a human standing on earth.

Time of day. UV levels are at their most intense at midday, when the sun is at its highest point in the sky. When the sun is at its highest point, the UV radiation has the shortest distance to travel through the atmosphere to earth. Contrarily, the sun's radiation must pass through the atmosphere at a more oblique angle during the early morning and late afternoon, and therefore UV intensity is greatly diminished at those times, which is why it's very difficult to make vitamin D in early morning or late afternoon sun.

Time of year. The angle of the sun changes with the seasons. This causes the intensity of the UV radiation to vary as well. UV intensity is greatest during the summer months.

Latitude. The sun's radiation is most intense at the equator, where the sun is directly overhead and its radiation has to travel the shortest distance through the earth's ozone layer. Therefore, at the equator, more UV radiation reaches the earth's surface from the sun. At higher latitudes the sun is lower in the sky and UV radiation has to travel a greater distance through more ozone to reach the earth's surface. This makes the UV radiation in middle and high latitudes less intense. People living in Edmonton, Canada, for example, cannot make any vitamin D in their skin during seven months of the year (from September through April). New Yorkers cannot make vitamin D during four months (from November through February).

Altitude. UV radiation is more intense at higher altitudes because there is less atmosphere to absorb it. When you are at higher altitudes, therefore, you are at greater risk of overexposure. A study we did with Dr. Edward Sauter comparing the body's vitamin D–making capacity at Everest Base Camp in the Himalayas (at an altitude of 17,700 feet) proved a person can make vitamin D year-round at such an elevation, but not at lower altitudes nearby. You could stand by the Taj Mahal in November and be deficient.

Weather conditions. The more clouds there are, the less UV radiation can penetrate to the earth's surface. However, UV radiation can penetrate cloud cover, which explains why you can still get sunburned on a hazy or overcast summer's day.

Reflection. Certain surfaces reflect UV radiation and increase its intensity even in shaded areas. Such surfaces include snow, sand, or water. With increased intensity comes a double dose.

Pollution. An increasing number of people live with pollution in their local atmosphere, from those in metropolitan settings like Los Angeles and Houston to those living in less densely populated areas where wind patterns move and trap polluted pockets of air in otherwise clean places. Because pollution can filter out UV radiation, less reaches the earth's surface. This may explain why vitamin D deficiency persists in Los Angeles and Atlanta, the two cities just on the border of latitudes where making vitamin D is relatively easy most of the year.

Think A for Aging and B for Burning

People get confused between UVA and UVB. It helps to think of the A-type radiation as contributing to premature wrinkles when exposure is excessive. Wind, pollution, and smoking also can damage the skin, especially if your exposure to these elements is extreme. Ironically, like melanoma, the wrinkled skin you see in many baby boomers may be a result of the advent of sunscreens in the 1960s. Why? These early sunscreens protected people from UVB radiation—which causes burning—enabling them to spend lengthy periods in the sun, but didn't shield them from deeply penetrating UVA.

At the time, UVA radiation wasn't thought to have any effect. We now know, however, that it is mostly the UVA radiation from sunshine that causes the damage responsible for wrinkles. Thus, early sunscreens contributed to premature wrinkling in people who used them because they could spend a long time in the sun without getting burned. In doing so, they were exposed to unnaturally large doses of UVA radiation, which penetrated deeply and had an added impact on their immune systems.

From UVB to Activated Vitamin D

The chain reaction starts when UVB rays hit the skin's surface, where, as I explained earlier, a precursor to cholesterol called 7-dehydrocholesterol (also called provitamin D_3 or 7-DHC) gets converted to previtamin D_3 right there in the upper layer of your skin. This compound then rapidly changes to vitamin D_3 that can be released from the skin cells and enter the bloodstream. This form is also called cholecalciferol, or vitamin D_3, and is the same form synthesized from sheep's lanolin for vitamin D_3 supplements. (I'll distinguish vitamin D_3 from D_2 shortly.) Vitamin D_3 is still biologically inactive until the liver takes it and creates the major circulating form, 25-vitamin D (alternatively called calcidiol).

But wait. Before vitamin D even gets to the liver to be changed into 25-vitamin D, some of it is going through your subcutaneous fat (the layer of fat just beneath your skin) and being stored. Vitamin D is fat soluble, so that's where it can be stored during winter months and released as needed. Just as a bear hibernates during the winter and restocks his fat cells during the warmer months from spring to fall, a human is meant to stock up on vitamin D during the sunny months and cash out those fat cells during those cold winter days.

The half-life of 25-vitamin D in your circulation is two to three weeks. Thus, one sensible sun exposure probably lasts you for at least one to two weeks.

I described earlier that before the main circulating form of vitamin D can carry out its functions, it must go through another gate—the kidneys. This is where 25-vitamin D becomes the active form, 1,25-vitamin D. And it is this active form that is responsible for regulating calcium metabolism and bone health. If you don't have adequate vitamin D, you can't use calcium. In fact, if you are deficient, you absorb no more than 10 percent to 15 percent of calcium in your diet or supplements. If you are vitamin D *insufficient*, you absorb less than 30 percent of dietary calcium. I'll define these parameters in detail below; in brief, being insufficient means you're technically not deficient but you still aren't meeting your body's full requirement.

The ability to absorb calcium is significant for everyone, and especially for people who are taking bone-health drugs like Fosamax (alendronate); Actonel (risedronate); Boniva (ibandronate); Reclast (zoledronic acid); or Forteo (teriparatide). Patients are often instructed to take calcium in addition to their drug treatment, but doctors fail to remind them about adequate vitamin D intake. Without the vitamin D available, the calcium you ingest is less useful. For all intents and purposes, that calcium is invisible to the body and its hungry bones. In chapter 9 I'll go into detail about the calcium connection and bone health and explain how vitamin D and calcium work together in synergy.

The Only Test for Vitamin D Status

So given all these different forms of vitamin D, you'd think the best one to test in a person would be the active form, right? Wrong.

It turns out that you cannot use your blood level of activated vitamin D, or even the form that moves from the skin cells to the liver, which is biologically inert, to arrive at an accurate measurement of vitamin D status. The major circulating form—25-vitamin D—is the most important vitamin D metabolite. It's the form I and all experts in my field recommend that doctors measure in patients to determine their vitamin D status. (On a lab report, you may see "serum 25(OH)D," which is the correct form.) Doctors are becoming more aware of the differences, but upwards of 20 percent of physicians still order the wrong test.

Vitamin D₂ versus Vitamin D₃: What's the Difference?

I get this question a lot. And I'm not surprised to find that many people believe that vitamin D_2 does nothing and it's all about vitamin D_3. My lab and others have just recently put this myth to bed.

The vitamin D that is made in your skin is vitamin D_3. Vitamin D_2, made from yeast and used for food fortification and supplements for more than sixty years, has been accused of being less effective than vitamin D_3 in maintaining 25-vitamin D levels. The lay press has promoted the idea that people should be careful about their vitamin D supplement and be sure that they are taking vitamin D_3 and not vitamin D_2. In 2008 I reported that when healthy young and middle-aged adults ingested

1,000 IU of vitamin D_2, they raised their blood levels of 25-vitamin D to the same extent as healthy adults ingesting 1,000 IU of vitamin D_3.

To be certain that vitamin D_2 wasn't enhancing the destruction of vitamin D_3, I designed the study to include a group who received 500 IU of vitamin D_2 and 500 IU of vitamin D_3 in the same capsule. My team and I observed that the blood levels of 25-vitamin D increased by ten nanograms (ng) per milliliter and was comparable to the level achieved by ingesting either 1,000 IU of vitamin D_2 or 1,000 IU of vitamin D_3. In other words, I demonstrated that vitamin D_2 is just as effective as vitamin D_3 and put to rest this long-established myth. Other labs have since confirmed this finding in children.

Because supplemental vitamin D_3 comes from an animal source (lanolin), vegans often avoid supplements or think that vitamin D_2 isn't good enough. Some assays report both sets of vitamin D, as in "25(OH)D_2" and "25(OH) D_3." This is fine; you just need the total 25(OH)D.

Most supplements sold today are vitamin D_3, but there's no harm in obtaining your supply from vitamin D_2, which is the ideal choice for vegans who don't want any animal sources in their supplements. Patients who are treated for severe vitamin D deficiency with high doses of prescribed vitamin D (to the tune of 50,000 IU per dose) receive D_2; it's currently the only FDA-approved vitamin D available to physicians to treat and prevent vitamin D deficiency at that dosage, and it works well. I have given patients this amount of vitamin D for up to six years without any toxicity (see chapter 10 for more about this).

What Constitutes a Deficiency?

My extensive studies have helped redefine what it means to be vitamin D deficient. Before one of my publications in the *Lancet* in 1998, vitamin D deficiency was defined as a having 25-vitamin D levels below 10 nanograms per milliliter. I demonstrated, however, that a blood level of twice that—20 nanograms per milliliter—is needed to prevent an unhealthy elevation in parathyroid hormone level. I and my colleagues, including Dr. Robert Heaney at Creighton University, established that

The Barometer of Vitamin D Status

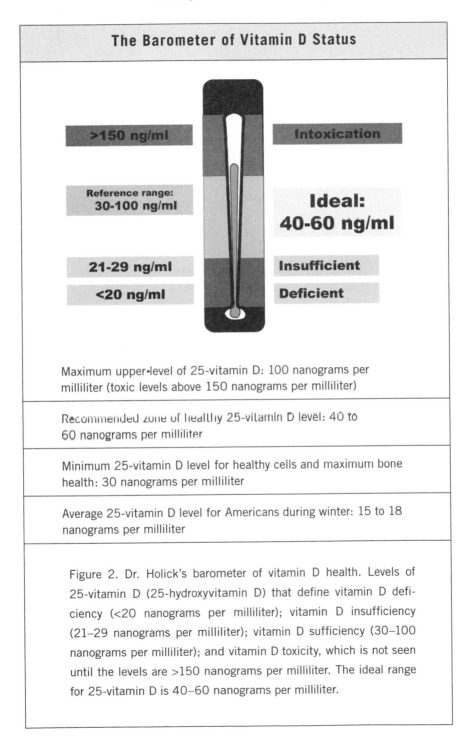

>150 ng/ml

Reference range:
30-100 ng/ml

21-29 ng/ml

<20 ng/ml

Intoxication

Ideal:
40-60 ng/ml

Insufficient

Deficient

Maximum upper-level of 25-vitamin D: 100 nanograms per milliliter (toxic levels above 150 nanograms per milliliter)

Recommended zone of healthy 25-vitamin D level: 40 to 60 nanograms per milliliter

Minimum 25-vitamin D level for healthy cells and maximum bone health: 30 nanograms per milliliter

Average 25-vitamin D level for Americans during winter: 15 to 18 nanograms per milliliter

Figure 2. Dr. Holick's barometer of vitamin D health. Levels of 25-vitamin D (25-hydroxyvitamin D) that define vitamin D deficiency (<20 nanograms per milliliter); vitamin D insufficiency (21–29 nanograms per milliliter); vitamin D sufficiency (30–100 nanograms per milliliter); and vitamin D toxicity, which is not seen until the levels are >150 nanograms per milliliter. The ideal range for 25-vitamin D is 40–60 nanograms per milliliter.

for every 100 IU of vitamin D ingested, the blood's level of 25-vitamin D goes up by 1 nanogram per milliliter. Don't worry about what that really means; the important point is that based on these observations, it is now recognized the international community now defines vitamin D deficiency as a having a 25-vitamin D level below 20 nanograms per milliliter. Vitamin D *insufficiency* is between 21 and 29 nanograms per milliliter. Ideally, you should aim to have a 25-vitamin D level of at least 30 nanograms per milliliter, and 100 nanograms per milliliter is safe.

Clearly, you're not going to see a vitamin D supplement that says "take this pill once a day and it will boost your 25-vitamin D levels to 40 nanograms per milliliter." And the sun won't stop shining once you've obtained enough to boost your vitamin D supplies. So how do you know how much you're getting and how that all translates to sufficient levels in your body?

That's where my three-step strategy comes in, which I'll take you through step by step in part II. But first, it's imperative to clear up a few common misconceptions about vitamin D that probably still have you scratching your head.

Your 25-vitamin D level is the barometer for your vitamin D status and is a summation of your dietary, supplemental, and sunlight sources of vitamin D. See chapter 7 for more about testing.

How Much Is Too Much?

Between 1987 and 1991, as many as forty-four thousand households in the Boston area were at risk of vitamin D "intoxication," the scientific word for overdosing. The culprit was home-delivered milk that had been overly fortified by one careless employee at a dairy company (rather than 400 IU of vitamin D per quart, there were up to 250,000 IU per quart). The index cases included a healthy seventy-six-year-old woman who died due to vitamin D intoxication, which can increase blood calcium and phosphate and calcify blood vessels and kidneys, and a young child who developed kidney failure, cases we reported in the *New England Journal of Medicine*. I helped uncover the source of the outbreak and put a stop to distribution of the tainted milk. The experience inspired me to conduct a study, published in the *New England Journal of Medicine* at the same time, that examined milk and infant-formula preparations. Milk rarely contains the amount of vitamin D stated on the label, but in most cases it's not overfortified—it's underfortified. Which is why my conclusion called for better monitoring of the fortification process. (We did, however, find that infant formulas contained at least the amount of vitamin D stated on the label.)

I'll give you one more example of an unusual case of vitamin D OD. At 7:00 one morning in the mid-1990s, I picked up the phone to hear an irate Florida lawyer accuse me of ruining his health by suggesting he take vitamin D supplements.

"Are you Dr. Holick?" he said.

"No." (I wasn't interested in talking to a lawyer at that hour. Who is?)

"Well, I know you're Dr. Holick because you're the only one there that early in the morning. And I'm gonna sue you."

"Why"? (Now I was interested.)

"Because I've been following your advice and I went on the Internet, bought some vitamin D, and now I've landed in the emergency room with vitamin D intoxication!"

No wonder I was at the top of his list of people to call and threaten with a lawsuit. Rather than hang up on the poor fellow and call my own lawyer, I kindly asked him to send his vitamin D to me so I could test it. I found it hard to believe he could be vitamin D intoxicated from the amount he believed he was taking.

Sure enough, the company had forgotten to dilute it. The two teaspoons a day he was taking in powder form weren't delivering a healthy 2,000 IU a day. He was taking *1,000,000* IU a day—plenty to cause vitamin D intoxication. He didn't sue me in the end, but rather he asked for my advice on how to recover from his vitamin D intoxication. He then took his complaint up with the supplement company, which quickly went out of business.

Sunlight destroys any excess vitamin D that your body makes, so you could never become vitamin D intoxicated from sun exposure. You would need to ingest more than 10,000 IU of vitamin D a day for at least half a year to even begin to worry about potential toxicity from supplements. Symptoms of toxicity include nausea, vomiting, loss of appetite, constipation, increased frequency of urination, increased thirst, disorientation, and weight loss.

Despite these two cases, vitamin D intoxication is extremely rare. And what I continually tell people is that there is absolutely no way to overdose on vitamin D through exposure to sunlight. The body, not surprisingly, has a way of regulating the amount required so that there's never an excess amount of vitamin D circulating in the bloodstream. If you expose yourself to the sun in a bathing suit for long enough to see a light pinkness twenty-four hours afterward, that's the equivalent of taking between 15,000 and 20,000 IU of vitamin D. For a white adult, that would be the equivalent of being exposed to sunlight in June at noon for about ten to fifteen minutes on a Cape Cod beach. Your body has a huge capacity to make vitamin D at any age. While aging does decrease levels of the provitamin D molecule responsible for making vitamin D in the skin, your body still has enough ingredients to make adequate vitamin D with adequate amounts of sunshine, even when you are ninety years old.

The Pros Beat the "Cons"

In 2002, an extraordinary amount of attention was being generated by an announcement concerning UV radiation and health. The federal government's National Toxicology Program had just announced that it had added ultraviolet radiation to the list of what it considers "known human carcinogens." As unfortunate as this move was by an agency of the U.S. Department of Health and Human Services, it perfectly encapsulates the misconceptions that prevail concerning sunlight and health.

The blanket statement that UV radiation is carcinogenic is confusing. As a friend of mine put it, saying that UV radiation causes cancer and should be avoided is akin to saying that water causes drowning, so don't drink water. It is misleading to place radiation on the list of carcinogens without saying that *overexposure*—not just exposure—is the problem. Too much of just about anything can be a problem—too much dietary fat, too much salt, and so on. There's a world of difference between moderation and excess. Just as we need a little fat and salt in our diet, we also need a little sun.

What's interesting when you read some of the finer print in the government's report on carcinogens is that it doesn't offer numbers that define parameters for safety levels. It states, "Listing of substances in the Report . . . does not establish that such substances present carcinogenic risks to individuals in their daily lives."

In my opinion, excluding this vital information makes the list of carcinogens pointless. The situation is similar to one in the 1980s, when the artificial sweetener saccharin was listed in the National Toxicology Program's Report on Carcinogens. Remember those warnings on soda can labels stating that the product had been shown to cause cancer in laboratory animals? Saccharin was removed from the list in 2002 because the amount needed to cause cancer even in lab animals—eight hundred cans of diet soda per rat!—was unrealistically large.

It's also important to keep in mind that carcinogens are present everywhere in nature. As scary as it may sound, there are known carcinogens in most food and drink, including tap water (chloroform), grain products (ethylene dibromide), bacon and other processed meats (nitrosamines), peanut butter (aflatoxin), brown mustard (allyl isothiocyanate), basil (estragole), mushrooms (hydrazines), beer and wine (ethyl alcohol), and, as I just pointed out, some diet sodas (saccharin). Here is what the American Council on Science and Health states about your chances of being free of all carcinogens: "No human diet can be free from all naturally occurring carcinogens or toxic substances. Indeed, it is hard to find any food that does not contain some harmful chemical that either occurs naturally or is produced during cooking or by microbial decomposition."

The point I'm making is that carcinogens are everywhere, including in natural substances that we need to survive. Just because something is natural doesn't mean we can consume or subject ourselves to unlimited amounts of it without suffering negative health consequences. Sugar, salt, and even water and oxygen are all dangerous when taken in excess. Despite the attention the tenth Report on Carcinogens received when UV radiation was put on the list, the inclusion means nothing more than that overexposure to sunlight may increase your risk of skin cancer. There are few people around who would deny this fact. But there are just as many people who have a hard time seeing UVB and health in the same column.

The Truth

How did we reach a point in our history when sun became something to be feared instead of revered? The simple answer lies in the fact that there are many billions of dollars to be made in emphasizing the only major medical downside of sun exposure (nonmelanoma skin cancer) and not much money to be made in promoting the sun's many benefits.

The decline of sunlight as a popular and successful treatment for a variety of diseases was initially hastened by major medical breakthroughs. It started with the discovery of penicillin in 1928. The success of this and other wonder drugs heralded the beginning of the era of pharmacology and saved the lives of millions. However, it also precipitated the eclipse of disciplines such as heliotherapy and photobiology, which appeared quaint and outdated by comparison. It wasn't long before people had been converted en masse to the idea that synthetic drugs were much more effective in preventing and curing most maladies that affect humankind than anything Mother Nature had to offer—a belief that largely prevails today.

Medicine has long known that, despite all the sun's benefits, a health downside of sun exposure is nonmelanoma skin cancer. In the 1920s, it was recognized that farmers in Europe developed skin cancer on their most sun-exposed areas—their ears, face, nose, and the backs of their hands. By 1937 the *American Journal of the Medical Sciences* published a report by Dr. Sigismund Peller of New York University that theorized how UV radiation could protect against the development of

more malignant cancers, albeit inducing benign and treatable skin cancer. Dr. Peller's population study of choice was a group of people famous
for its time in the sun by virtue of the job: the U.S. Navy. Compared to
age-matched controls, the rate of skin cancer in the U.S. Navy was eight
times higher, while the total number of deaths from other cancers was
60 percent *less* than in the civilian population. And in 1941, the first
issue of the *Journal of Cancer* put the issue in perfect perspective, stating that an increased risk of nonmelanoma skin cancer was one of the
prices to be paid for a *decreased* risk of cancer of the prostate, breast,
and colon. Studies like this were later repeated, confirming the same
conclusion. A look at navy personnel again, this time over a ten-year
period in the 1970s and 1980s, revealed the same pattern. People who
worked in jobs that had them outdoors had the lowest rates of melanoma.
Those who took mostly to the indoors for work, on the other hand, had
the highest incidence of melanoma.

Unfortunately, in the past quarter century, the relationship between
sunlight and skin cancer has been blown out of proportion. The major
culprits are the cosmetic wing of the pharmaceutical industry and what
I consider to be some unenlightened dermatologists. In the 1960s and
1970s, as the leisure culture expanded and people were spending more
time outdoors, the "cosmeceutical" industry developed antisunburn
creams that gave the user a false sense of security and encouraged excessive sun exposure.

Antisunburn products began making extraordinary amounts of
money for the companies that produced them. Although the products
were initially introduced to prevent sunburn, they soon were being can-
nily marketed to prevent skin cancer. There is an important role for
modern sunscreens in preventing skin cancer, and people should control
sun exposure in the same way they watch how much salt, sugar, and fat
they eat and how much alcohol they drink. However, the sophisticated
and aggressive "educational" campaigns funded by the cosmeceutical
industry have created an antisunshine hysteria that is detrimental to our
health because it converts people into sunphobes by convincing them
that no amount of unprotected sun exposure is sensible or important for
health.

So desperate is the antisun lobby to convince you of the dangers of the sun (so that you will buy its products year-round) that its representatives will tell you with a straight face that if it's February in Boston and you're planning to walk to the corner store to buy a quart of milk or sit outside on your lunch break, you should wear sunscreen. This message has recently been taken to the extreme by a New York City dermatologist on a popular morning TV station suggesting that you should wear sunscreen even indoors because fluorescent lamps can damage your skin and cause cancer. This is wrongheaded and alarmist. Even on the sunniest February day, the sun isn't strong enough in New England, New York, or San Francisco to increase your risk of skin cancer significantly. That said, it still has plenty of UVA radiation that can damage your skin's elasticity and your immune system. This is but one example of the kind of inaccurate information the antisun lobby puts out to alarm people. In so doing, it convinces people of the need for its products and services year-round indoors and out.

The scare tactics of the cosmeceutical industry have been embraced by most of the dermatology profession. These groups have worked in concert and have frightened the daylights out of people—or, more accurately, frightened people out of the daylight. To put the dangers of skin cancer in context, it's worthwhile to look at some statistics. Nonmelanoma skin cancer, which may be caused by long-term sun exposure, has an extremely low death rate. Fewer than 0.5 percent of people who develop nonmelanoma skin cancer die; nonmelanoma skin cancer claims 1,200 lives a year in the United States. Compare that with diseases that can be prevented by regular sun exposure.

Colon and breast cancers, which are two of the most common types of cancer and which may be prevented by regular sun exposure, have mortality rates of 20 percent to 65 percent and kill nearly 100,000 Americans annually. Osteoporosis, a bone disease that can be mitigated by regular sun exposure, is endemic, affecting 25 million Americans. Every year, 1.5 million Americans with osteoporosis suffer bone fractures, which can be fatal when the person is elderly; 300,000 of those are hip fractures, and 20 percent of patients (or 60,000 individuals) will die within the first year after such a break. When I think of the monetary costs, not to mention the emotional and psychological toll, related to treating the diseases and injuries related to vitamin D deficiency, the fire in my belly to keep talking about all this data reignites.

Some fifty thousand to seventy thousand Americans die prematurely each year because of insufficient UV exposure, compared with the nine thousand to ten thousand deaths in the United States due to skin cancer—skin cancer that can be prevented and treated when detected early.

Though rare, melanomas are by far the most dangerous form of skin cancer, and, if left untreated, they are often fatal. Eighty percent of all skin cancer fatalities are attributed to this type of cancer. However — and this is a critical point—there is no credible scientific evidence that moderate sun exposure causes melanomas. In chapter 8, I will clear up the confusion surrounding the relationship between sun exposure and skin cancer, confusion that the media doesn't seem able to unravel and the antisun lobby has a vested interest in maintaining.

The antisun lobby also plays on people's fear of developing wrinkles—a growing concern in our youth-obsessed culture. It's true that sun exposure causes the skin to age prematurely, but it is possible to take advantage of the benefits of sun exposure while minimizing wrinkles.

So why has no one stood up to the antisun lobby and said, "Hey, wait a minute, for too long you've exaggerated the dangers of sun exposure and ignored the fact that human beings need sunlight to live"? Well, I have! The problem is, whenever anyone challenges the antisun-coalition doctrine that sun exposure does nothing but cause skin cancer and wrinkles—usually by publishing a new study that demonstrates a positive link between sunlight and disease prevention—this news is drowned out by another well-funded round of disinformation about the hazards of sun exposure. The bibliography at the end of the book lists many of the published studies that show the beneficial association between the vitamin D you get from sunlight and many areas of health.

It's difficult to get the facts out because there is no sun lobby. Sunshine is free, after all, so there's not much money to be made extolling its virtues. Clearly there's a lot of work to be done to promote the importance of UV radiation for all-around health. This book should help alter public perception of the role of sunlight in our lives. Certainly I hope it helps you make more informed decisions about your relationship to sunshine and human well-being. Increasing numbers of scholarly articles are being published that address the beneficial relationship between UVB radiation and health—to the point that even my beloved American Academy of Dermatology, the very institution that has criticized my advice in the past, is showing signs of weakening in the face of so many indisputable papers from the most esteemed campuses in the world.

The very day I wrote this page, another study emerged declaring that one in seven American teenagers is vitamin D deficient, including fully half of black teenagers. Overweight teens are twice as likely to be deficient as teens of healthy weight, and girls have twice the risk of boys. These are sobering statistics, especially against the backdrop of our climbing obesity epidemic. The link between obesity and vitamin D deficiency poses an added challenge because it's more difficult for obese individuals to push their levels of vitamin D up.

Depending on what kind of skin you have, where you live, and what time of year it is, you need sun exposure in varying amounts to maintain adequate levels of vitamin D. It is true that there are some drawbacks to excessive sun exposure, and I examine these in depth in later chapters of this book. However, as you will see, the drawbacks of sun exposure pale in comparison with the health benefits.

Let's put the pros and cons of sunlight into perspective with an analogy. Exercise is another example of something that has both benefits and drawbacks but that is, on the whole, good for you. Everyone knows that exercising is good. It prevents a variety of chronic illnesses and makes you look and feel better. But if you exercise too much, or if you have certain predisposing risk factors—flat feet or a faulty backhand—then you may develop overuse conditions such as Achilles tendonitis or lateral epicondylitis ("tennis elbow"). Every year, people die of heart attacks while running or lifting weights. Nevertheless, no self-respecting doctor would take the position that exercise is unhealthy. Most doctors will tell you to take certain precautions when exercising, but none would ever advise you not to be active.

The same goes for sun exposure. Sunlight is not unhealthy. Precautions do need to be taken, but a regular, moderate amount of unprotected sun exposure is absolutely necessary for good health—as you will come to discover as you turn the pages of this book.

CHAPTER 3

Hard Bodies

The magic of D on muscle and bone health

When you think of old age, the words *frail* and *weak* may come to mind. You might picture a doddering woman or man hunched over a cane with loose, crepe-like skin, thin threads of hair, and a reedy voice. What you don't see is a well-postured individual with a lot of toned muscles and signs of physical strength. If this person once had the physique of an athlete or the carriage of a model, it is evident only in old photographs. Few people think about the role muscle mass plays in the aging process, and how muscle works in tandem with bone to keep us agile, able-bodied, and above all, young.

The average American gains one pound of body weight each year after the age of twenty-five, yet loses one third to one half a pound of muscle. Although a fraction of a pound of muscle mass may seem minuscule, it actually adds up to be quite remarkable—translating to about a 1 percent to 2 percent loss of strength each year. Muscle strength typically peaks between ages twenty and thirty and then gradually decreases, resulting in the majority of people experiencing a 30 percent loss in overall strength by age seventy. Of course, this can be partially offset if one is diligent about trying to maintain and continue to build muscle mass through exercise and, in particular, strength training. But for many people, age brings a combination of unique circumstances and physical conditions that can infringe on the quest to retain muscle mass. So the decline continues, and with this loss of muscle strength we become even less active because daily activities become more difficult and exhausting. All of this exacerbates the muscle loss and magnifies a person's overall frailty.

The reason strength training gets so much attention in fitness circles is that it supports lean muscle mass and can help you to increase muscle mass, strength, and bone health. The muscles you engage when you lift a weight put pressure on your bones, forcing them to get stronger. In fact, recent studies have shown that loss of bone density may be a better predictor of death from atherosclerosis (hardening of the arteries) than cholesterol levels. There are other benefits, too. Strength training is an effective antidepressant and can even improve sleep quality.

We don't normally hear about people losing out on life or dying from muscle loss. But we do hear a lot about bone loss and osteoporosis, especially with regard to women after menopause. Pharmaceutical companies have started marketing their osteoporosis drugs directly to consumers, promising to help women maintain bone density and even reverse bone loss. Two facts to note: (1) one of these aggressively marketed drugs has no impact on the risk of hip fractures; it only reduces spinal fractures, which are far less life threatening than hip breaks; and (2) more than half of women taking these drugs (58 percent) have been shown to be vitamin D deficient or insufficient. One can markedly reduce the chance of hip fracture through adequate levels of calcium and vitamin D.

Earlier I touched upon bone diseases such as rickets, osteomalacia, and osteoporosis and their association with vitamin D. Let's take a closer look at these conditions and then loop back to muscle health. You'll come to see just how critical vitamin D is in your body's musculoskeletal structure and how your own version of "old age" may have everything to do with maintaining your vitamin D levels.

Growing Up and Boning Up

The thought of bones often conjures scenes from archaeological digs or a cemetery. Your bones, though, are living things made up of substances that are continually breaking down and being rebuilt. This process is known as remodeling.

Every year, 20 percent to 40 percent of your skeleton is renewed. Children's bodies make new bone faster than they break down existing bone, which causes bone mass to increase. People reach their peak bone mass in their twenties. However, in the late thirties, the body begins to break down more bone than it makes. This decrease is slight; normal bone loss is only about 0.3 percent to 0.5 percent per year. The result of this slow loss is that the skeleton becomes less dense and more fragile. The process accelerates the older you get. After menopause, women lose bone density at a rate of 2 percent to 4 percent every year. Men lose 1 percent to 2 percent after the age of sixty.

It goes without saying that if you are trying to ensure the health of your bones, the goal should be to build bone mass when you are young and to maintain it when you get past the age when bone remodeling is at its peak. If you do this, chances are you won't have problems with your bones later in life. But if you don't build bone mass when you are young, and if you lose bone mass at an excessive rate after the peak bone-building age, your bones can get more porous and brittle (osteoporosis, a painless disease), which means they can break more easily. If the bone-rebuilding process itself is compromised, you may have symptoms such as persistent pain and bone deformity (osteomalacia or rickets).

How can you build bone mass when you are young and maintain it when you are older? The answer to both questions is the same: be active and get enough calcium in your diet. When we emphasize calcium intake for bone health, the importance of vitamin D is often ignored. But vitamin D is like the yeast in a recipe for bread. You can't make bone without vitamin D available. And it all starts in your parathyroid glands and intestine.

The opposing processes of bone resorption (the dissolving of existing bone tissue) and formation (the filling of the resulting small cavities with new bone tissue) are well regulated so that an adult's total mass of bone tissue normally remains nearly constant, but it's constantly being broken down and replaced such that 20 percent to 40 percent of an adult's skeleton is remodeled every year. In an infant's first year of life, almost 100 percent of his or her skeleton is replaced.

A number of factors affect bone development, growth, and repair, including hormones, exercise, and vitamin D synthesis. Vitamin D is necessary for proper absorption of calcium in the small intestine, from which it can move to your skeleton via your bloodstream and be deposited in the bones to given them their strength—rather like a cement. When vitamin D is absent, calcium is poorly absorbed, which compromises the bone-remodeling process—not enough bone is made to replace the bone that is broken down. The constant breakdown and replacement of bone that occurs throughout your life is spurred largely by parathyroid hormone, which is released from your parathyroid glands, which sit on the upper and lower poles of your thyroid. Without enough calcium moving to your bones thanks to vitamin D's presence, that delicate dance between bone breakdown and bone creation can become imbalanced. In other words, you can eat as much calcium-rich food, drink as much milk, and take as many calcium supplements as you want to, but if you don't have enough vitamin D in your body, you won't be able to effectively absorb that calcium for your bones. And you won't be able to outpace the breakdown of bones, leading to serious bone-related conditions.

So why is calcium so critical? The intercellular collagen matrix of bone tissue needs a considerable amount of calcium hydroxyapatite to have normal bone mineralization. It is estimated that a person who is vitamin D deficient will absorb only about one third to one half as much calcium as he or she would with a healthy vitamin D status. Without enough vitamin D to help your bones absorb calcium—or without enough calcium itself—your bones don't remodel properly. This can happen at any age. And it's not just about bone health. Low calcium absorption triggers a cascade of physiological problems, as calcium is important for most metabolic functions and neuromuscular activities.

Can Osteoporosis Be Averted Despite Advanced Age?

The most commonly known bone disease is osteoporosis, which is characterized by porous, brittle, and weak bones. Vitamin D deficiency can cause osteoporosis, and it can make it worse. Even when people are consuming enough calcium, numerous studies have shown that they still will not build and maintain bone mass if they are deficient in vitamin D. And even more studies have shown that people who suffer from osteoporosis often have vitamin D deficiency.

As I've been reiterating, not getting enough vitamin D doesn't just affect your bones in old age. If you don't get enough vitamin D during those early years when it's crucial to build bone mass—up until your thirties—you won't establish the bone mass you need to keep your bones strong when you naturally break down more of the bone structure than you can make. Men do get osteoporosis, but women are at much greater risk. Because women have less testosterone, they have less muscle mass (this also explains why women have a harder time building and maintaining muscle mass, as testosterone factors heavily into one's muscle mass). Women, in fact, start out with lower bone mass and tend to live longer; they also experience a sudden drop in estrogen at menopause that accelerates bone loss. At the beginning of menopause, women can lose as much as 3 percent to 4 percent of bone mass every year. Slender, small-framed women are particularly at risk. Men who have low levels of the male hormone testosterone are also at increased risk. Doctors can detect early signs of osteoporosis with a simple, painless bone density test (densitometry).

You are at especially high risk of vitamin D deficiency–related osteoporosis if you are predisposed to vitamin D deficiency. There is one exception when comparing the risks of vitamin D deficiency and osteoporosis. Although people of African descent living in higher latitudes are at higher risk of vitamin D deficiency because their bodies don't convert sunlight into vitamin D as easily as races with fairer skin, they do not appear to be at a higher risk of osteoporosis than those with fairer skin. The reason for this is that people of African genetic lineage tend to start with 9 percent to 15 percent denser bones than Caucasian people. However, chronic vitamin D deficiency will overcome this natural protection and cause African Americans to suffer increased loss of bone density and risk of fracture.

An indication of the importance of vitamin D on the bone density of seniors was found in a study my colleagues and I did of senior citizens living in Maine, which showed that they lost 3 percent to 4 percent of their bone mass in the fall and winter and regained it in the spring and summer months. Obviously, the most serious problem associated with osteoporosis is fractures. As noted previously, osteoporosis is responsible for 1.5 million fractures each year, most notably fractures of the vertebrae (causing the hunched appearance often seen in elderly women and painful sciatica due to nerve compression in the lower back), ribs, wrists, and hips. Hip fractures tend to be crippling and are sometimes fatal. Osteoporosis-related fractures are more common during the winter months, when muscles tend to be weaker and there's an increased risk of falling. Unless a person remains active during the winter months, thus keeping up muscle mass and bone strength, there's a greater likelihood of falling and breaking bones. A vitamin D deficiency could worsen the situation, since UVB-absent winter months require adequate storage of vitamin D for use and vitamin D supplementation.

Because there is no pain until a fracture occurs, osteoporosis is known as the silent threat. Numerous studies have shown that vitamin D—usually in conjunction with calcium—is an effective treatment for increasing or maintaining bone density and preventing fractures associated with osteoporosis. Finnish researchers found that 341 elderly people (mostly women ages seventy-five and older) who were given vitamin D injections experienced fewer fractures than 458 people who did not receive the supplements. A French study of 3,270 elderly women showed 43 percent fewer hip fractures in participants who were given an 800 IU vitamin D supplement every day and 800 milligrams of calcium than in those participants who were given a placebo. A study of a less high-risk group was done by Dr. Bess Dawson-Hughes and her colleagues in the Boston area when 391 men and women ages sixty-five and older were given either a 700 IU vitamin D supplement or a placebo. The results showed that the participants who were given the supplement sustained half as many fractures as the placebo group and experienced significant bone density increases.

What Is Bone Densitometry?

Bone densitometry is a specialized kind of X-ray. Bone densitometry cal-culates how much the X-ray beams are absorbed when passing through bones. The amount of X-ray beams absorbed reveals to doctors the density of the bones being studied. (Density refers to the amount of calcium in the bones. Here's a bit of trivia that few people know: the reason bones look white on an X-ray or appear more dense in bone-mineral-density tests is that the atomic weight of calcium is at least two to forty times greater than that of hydrogen, oxygen, and carbon, which make up the soft tissues and surrounding collagen. Hence, the "heavy" calcium is absorbing more of the X-rays and showing up more brightly.) Bone densitometry may be done on the bones of the spine, hip, or wrist. Vitamin D deficiency causes more bone loss in the wrist and hip than in the spine. The result of a densitometry test is known as a T-score and is calculated based on how different your bones are from the bone density of a normal young person of your race and gen-der. A score greater than −2.5 puts you in the category of having osteopo-rosis. Sometimes, however, this test isn't useful. A bone density test done on a person who has a compression fracture of the spine, for example, will show bones that appear to be dense because of the compression and the pile of calcium in that compression. In this case, you can't evaluate the true condition of the bone, much less distinguish good bone from brittle bone.

How Drugs to Treat Osteoporosis Work

In 1995, Fosamax became the first medication in a class of drugs called bisphosphonates to come on the market and be approved for treating osteoporosis. Since then, other drugs in the same class have fol-lowed. Bisphosphonates affect the bone-remodeling cycle, which, again, is the body's balancing act between breaking bone down and form-ing new bone. In a healthy individual, the bone breakdown-formation process is equal, so you form new bone as fast as you dissolve old bone. But when these two parts of the cycle are not in sync, which can happen due to disease or missing ingredients like vitamin D to help complete the cycle, you eventually have osteoporosis.

Bisphosphonates essentially slow or stop the bone-dissolving portion of the remodeling cycle, thus allowing new bone formation to catch up with bone resorption. These drugs have been found to reduce spinal fractures by as much as 60 percent over three years and hip fractures by as much as 50 percent. The most dramatic results are seen in the first three to five years of taking the medication, and smaller improvements are made for up to a total of ten years. If a patient stops taking the drug, however, he or she will begin to lose the bone that was initially regained.

These drugs are far from perfect, however. They can be costly, and they are not side-effect free for everyone. Some patients experience gastrointestinal problems that can be too much to bear. These side effects explain why patients are asked to sit in an upright position, which prevents the drug from moving back up into the esophagus and causing irritation. The drug is not absorbed if food is around, which is why patients need to avoid drinking or eating for thirty minutes following the drug's administration, or for sixty minutes after taking Boniva.

Fosamax (alendronate), Actonel (risedronate), and Boniva (ibandronate) are approved for both the prevention and treatment of postmenopausal osteoporosis; however, whereas Fosamax and Actonel have been shown to reduce hip and vertebral fractures, Boniva has only been approved by the FDA to reduce the risk of spinal fractures. Miacalcin (calcitonin-salmon) and Evista (raloxifene) offer protection against vertebral fractures but not hip fractures. Forteo (teriparatide) actually stimulates bone formation and significantly reduces vertebral and non-vertebral fracture risk. This medication is actually not a bisphosphonate. It's a manmade parathyroid hormone used in postmenopausal women, and in men who are at high risk for fracture and who have not responded to bisphosphonate therapy; long-term use (greater than two years) is not currently encouraged. A newer bisphosphonate called Reclast (zoledronic acid solution) has since joined the market. This once-a-year treatment is given intravenously in a fifteen-minute procedure so that it bypasses the gastrointestinal tract. Also a bisphosphonate, Reclast is said to increase bone strength and reduce fractures in the hip, spine, wrist, arm, leg, and rib.

Despite our access to these powerful drugs today, in no way do they replace the need to ensure your calcium intake is sufficient and your vitamin D levels are strong. These drugs can only work as well as their target body's supply of the raw ingredients that participate in the bone-formation process. Most of the studies done with bisphosphonates that reported good results required calcium and vitamin D supplementation.

These drugs aside, it helps to remember that vitamin D supplementation has been shown to help reduce the likelihood of falling by more than 20 percent, which is important for patients with already compromised bone health. In a randomized, double-blind trial, treatment with vitamin D plus calcium daily for three months reduced the risk of falling by 49 percent compared with calcium alone among elderly women in long-stay geriatric care. In my own studies with Dr. Douglas Kiel and his group, we've shown a 72 percent decrease in the risk of falling on 800 IU of vitamin D for five months. And keep in mind that vitamin D has a broad range of activities beyond its role in calcium metabolism and bone health. Vitamin D has a say in numerous illnesses—cancer, rheumatoid arthritis, multiple sclerosis, type 1 diabetes, type 2 diabetes, heart disease, dementia, schizophrenia, and hypertension—many of which come to define a person's quality of life and life span.

A fifty-year-old white female has a 40 percent risk of experiencing an osteoporotic fracture in her lifetime. If she minimizes her bone loss, however, and can postpone bone loss by ten years, her risk of fracturing a bone goes down by as much as 50 percent later in life.

Why Osteomalacia Is So Painful

Bone problems don't just crop up late in life after they've had time to brew over the years unnoticed. There's somewhat of an expectation that an elderly person will have weaker bones than a younger counterpart. Age does, in fact, decrease bone resilience. A fifty-year-old and a seventy-year-old with the same bone density will have very different risk for fractures. The seventy-year-old will have a two to four times greater risk of fracture.

Age-related bone issues aside, few people think about serious bone-related disorders in younger people, which can make for more challenging diagnoses when doctors can't put their finger on a diagnosis for a patient complaining of general aches and pains. If you have bone pain and your muscles ache and feel weak, you may have a vitamin D deficiency–related condition I described earlier called osteomalacia. Osteomalacia is frequently described as "softening of the bones." This is slightly misleading. Osteomalacia is a condition in which the bones don't harden properly during the building phase. A lack of vitamin D is the most common cause of osteomalacia.

Unlike osteoporosis, which is often referred to as a silent disease because there are no symptoms until a fracture occurs, the chief characteristic of osteomalacia is severe, unrelenting, deep bone pain. This pain is felt in the bones of the arms, legs, chest, spine, and/or pelvis. Usually there is tenderness of the bones when the doctor pushes down even lightly on the area, and this can be misinterpreted as a trigger point for fibromyalgia. The pain from osteomalacia is a result of the unhardened, Jell-O-like bone matter pressing outward against the periosteum, which is the nerve-filled fibrous sheath that covers the bones. People with osteomalacia often complain of throbbing, aching bone pain and muscle aches and weakness.

Osteomalacia most severely affects sufferers during the winter months, when lack of vitamin D production is most pronounced. Often the pain associated with osteomalacia is constant, pounding, and severe. As a result, it can interfere with daily activities and sleep. Muscle aches and weakness are also common and come and go unexpectedly. This pain can increase the risk of injuries from falling. If you have osteomalacia that continues unabated, it will weaken your bones and predispose you to fractures, especially of the lower spine, hip, and wrist.

How do we test for osteomalacia? X-rays and bone density tests aren't effective diagnostic tools because they cannot distinguish between osteomalacia and osteoporosis. If my patient complains of the characteristic symptoms of this condition and a physical examination reveals bone pain when I press down lightly on the breastbone (sternum), the outside of the shin of the lower leg, and the forearms, then I diagnose that person with vitamin D deficiency–related osteomalacia and initiate intensive vitamin D therapy, including moderate sun exposure in spring, summer, and fall. To confirm the diagnosis, I order a blood test to measure the serum level of 25-vitamin D, the most accurate gauge of a person's vitamin D status. I prescribe 50,000 IU of vitamin D$_2$ once a week for eight weeks. After two months, I test the patient's blood again to make sure the vitamin D deficiency shows signs of improvement. If it does not, I prescribe another eight-week course of 50,000 IU doses of vitamin D$_2$ once a week; obese patients may need twice as much to raise levels of vitamin D. Usually the therapy I prescribe resolves the condition, though it's not an overnight success story. It can take up to a full year before the patient feels better and levels of vitamin D are consistently sufficient. Your doctor can get more information on how to treat and prevent vitamin D deficiency on my Web site, www.drholicksdsolution.com.

Countless studies have reported great results from treating osteomalacia patients with a protocol to up vitamin D levels. Restoring 25-vitamin D levels to normal in patients with this condition has resulted in complete resolution of pain, though I'll admit that the healing process takes time and patience. It can take months or years to develop osteomalacia, and it may take just as long to overcome it.

Can Fibromyalgia Be Disguised Osteomalacia?

Muscle pain, bone aches, feelings of weakness, and fatigue that just won't quit. These are the hallmarks of fibromyalgia. And osteomalacia. Are they the same thing? There has been a dramatic increase in various conditions with vague symptoms and no proven way to diagnose them. Among these conditions is fibromyalgia (sometimes known by the names fibrositis, chronic muscle pain syndrome, psychogenic rheumatism, or tension myalgias). Fibromyalgia was unknown until twenty years ago. There is no specific test to confirm that a person has fibromyalgia. It is a diagnosis of exclusion. That is, when everything else has been ruled out, this must be what's wrong.

Many people who are told they have fibromyalgia actually have osteomalacia. When someone shows up at a doctor's office with fuzzy symptoms of aching bone pain and muscle weakness, the physician is usually not aware that these are symptoms of vitamin D deficiency. Thus, the patient's vitamin D status is not tested. If it were, doctors would discover that many of the people with these symptoms are vitamin D deficient. Between 40 percent and 60 percent of the people who come to my clinic having been diagnosed with fibromyalgia or chronic fatigue or written off as having depression actually have vitamin D deficiency–related osteomalacia. These patients can be successfully treated with vitamin D supplementation and exposure to sunlight.

Between 40 percent and 60 percent of the people who come to my clinic having been diagnosed with fibromyalgia or chronic fatigue actually have vitamin D deficiency–related osteomalacia. Many have also been written off as victims of depression.

A study of Muslim women living in Denmark who had muscle pain and symptoms consistent with the symptoms of fibromyalgia revealed that 88 percent of them were vitamin D deficient. Women in this culture tend to get little sunlight because they spend a lot of time at home and when they go out are obliged to cover themselves entirely. Similar observations have been made in Saudi Arabia, Qatar, and the United Arab Emirates.

Other studies have also demonstrated how a misdiagnosis as simple as missing a vitamin D deficiency can lead to an exhaustive process of elimination that keeps patients in pain and prolongs their corrective treatment. Dr. Gregory A. Plotnikoff of the University of Minnesota Medical School reported in 2003 that among 150 children and adults aged ten to sixty-five years old who presented to an emergency department complaining of nonspecific muscular skeletal aches and pains, 93 percent were vitamin D deficient. These patients were initially given a wide variety of diagnoses, including degenerative joint disease, chronic depression (technically called dysthymia), chronic fatigue syndrome, arthritis, and, of course, fibromyalgia. They were also given a wide range of treatments; young women were sent home on over-the-counter NSAIDs (nonsteroidal anti-inflammatory drugs, e.g., Aleve) whereas an older African American gentleman (fifty-eight years old) was sent home on a narcotic, among many other powerful drugs. Dr. Plotnikoff was stunned to find no 25-vitamin D at all in five patients who had been told their pain was "all in their head."

In a remarkable case solved by doctors at the University of Connecticut, a seventy-eight-year-old man with severe muscle weakness and muscle twitches was suspected to have amyotrophic lateral sclerosis (ALS, commonly known as Lou Gehrig's disease). This was a misdiagnosis. All of the elderly man's symptoms disappeared after his underlying vitamin D deficiency was identified and corrected.

A Pain in the Back

Back pain is the most common neurological complaint in North America, second only to headache. In America, more than $50 billion is spent each year on treatment, much of it to no avail if a specific cause is not found. Chronic back pain is often progressive, and many sufferers never get diagnosed with anything specific to target in curing the back pain forever. Is there a link between some of these cases and vitamin D deficiency?

An article published in the *Journal of the American Board of Family Medicine* in 2008 looked at six cases where patients had experienced either chronic back pain or failed back surgery. After raising their 25-vitamin D levels from a state of insufficiency or deficiency to sufficiency, they showed significant improvement. Some were actually cured of their back ailments entirely, prompting the author of the article, Dr. Gerry Schwalfenberg, to call for more attention to possible vitamin D deficiencies in patients who complain of back pain.

Rickets Revisited

Let me add a few more facts about rickets, also known as pediatric osteomalacia, that I left out earlier. The sad fact about bone-development problems in children is that they usually aren't detected early enough to thwart some of the lifelong side effects. In adults, no matter how bad the pain, there are no visible symptoms of osteomalacia. In children whose bones are still growing, however, bones that don't harden properly may bend under the weight of the child's body due to gravity as the child begins to stand and walk. The most prominent signs of rickets are legs that bend inward or outward and a sunken chest with rivetlike bone protrusions up and down both sides of the breast. The ends of the bones of the arms and legs may be wider than normal.

In addition to these visible deformities, children with rickets experience bone pain and muscle weakness but may not be able to successfully convey their pain. Rickets was first identified in Europe in the mid-1600s, and, as you know by now, it became a major problem during the Industrial Revolution. Doctors of the era were dismayed to find widespread bone deformation in urban youngsters that was unknown in European farm kids or even the poorest children of Asia and Africa. Dr. Jedrzej Sniadecki of Poland determined that rickets was caused by lack of sunlight. European cities were a maze of dark alleyways where the sun did not penetrate, and overhead the skies were clouded with heavy pollution. Furthermore, many children of this period were forced to work all day in factories.

It wasn't until the 1920s that Drs. Alfred Hess and Lester Unger—working from the research of Dr. Sniadecki and Dr. Huldschinsky—finally got people's attention when they demonstrated in New York that sunlight was the magic bullet to cure rickets. Even though a handful of scientists and doctors had realized decades earlier that UV radiation from the sun was important for health and could cure rickets, it took a long time for the evidence to catch on in general circles and be accepted.

Soon after sunlight became the standard treatment for rickets (artificial sunlight from mercury arc lamps was also used), scientists discovered it was possible to fortify milk with vitamin D, and governments in Europe and North America sanctioned the fortification of milk and other foods. (As an aside, Dr. Harry Steenboch at the University of Wisconsin–Madison demonstrated that you could irradiate foods to impart anti-rachitic activity. This is the same lab that Dr. DeLuca took over after Dr. Steenboch retired.) Rickets, for the time being, was effectively eradicated. However, in the 1950s, there was an outbreak of elevated calcium in infants in the United Kingdom that caused permanent brain damage. Government officials unjustly attributed it to the overfortification of milk since vitamin D fortification was unregulated. Although overfortified milk was never proven to be the reason, European governments moved quickly to pass laws prohibiting the fortification of milk or any other food products with this vitamin. And rickets has again become a significant health problem in children living in cramped European urban communities such as London, Glasgow, and Paris. Sweden and Finland, however, do now fortify milk, margarine, and cereals, while other European countries only fortify margarine and cereals.

The United States has seen a resurgence of rickets in the last few years. This has motivated the American Academy of Pediatrics to voice its concern and reconsider its recommended daily vitamin D intake for children and adolescents. Because the disease had become so rare, doctors are not required by law to report it, so no national statistics are available. Doctors trained in an era that hasn't seen rickets are also not up to speed on spotting and treating it. That may change in the near future.

The main reasons for the reemergence of this condition are the increase in breast-feeding of infants (human milk contains almost no vitamin D) and the decline in young children's exposure to natural sunlight. Breast-feeding is important for a child's health, but it is important that both infant and mother take a vitamin D supplement, which I'll cover in chapter 10.

Although the incidence of rickets among American children is still extremely low, it is a growing problem. Parents need to be vigilant about their children's diet and lifestyle. The foundation of treatment for rickets is restoring the child's vitamin D status. Bracing and sometimes surgery may be necessary to correct skeletal deformities that have occurred. Once a child has been affected by rickets, there's no turning back from many of its ravages. He or she may never grow to become as tall or as strong as programmed by genetics. And the child's risk of other diseases, such as certain cancers, type 1 diabetes, and multiple sclerosis, is also markedly increased. Not a great way to start a long, healthy life—especially given the fact this disease is completely preventable with adequate vitamin D and calcium. Even a child who suffers from less severe vitamin D deficiency will be held back from reaching his or her full development and peak bone mass. If the child continues on through adulthood with below-adequate levels of vitamin D, he or she will likely experience a hormonal imbalance called secondary hyperparathyroidism, which then accelerates bone turnover and progressive bone loss—all of this leading to an increased risk for osteomalacia and osteoporosis. Osteoporosis, by the way, can start decades before "old age"; people as young as twentysomething have been diagnosed with this debilitating condition. (In 2002, a University of Arkansas study revealed that 2 percent of college-age women already have osteoporosis, and a further 15 percent have sustained significant losses in bone density.)

A long-term bone-health study of U.S. children is now being done in response to this resurgence in rickets, and researchers are concerned that widespread osteoporosis may be waiting for this younger generation in adulthood. But some researchers are just as concerned about the less well-known effects that low vitamin D levels may have on these children later in life. Dr. Cedric Garland, who has been researching vitamin D for over twenty years, estimates that we could prevent 75 percent of cancers by getting everyone's vitamin D blood level into an optimal range. (More on this cancer connection is coming up in the next chapter.)

Leaps and Bounds

If you had to let one thing go in life, which would it be: muscle or bone? Hard choice to make, isn't it? These two tissues work in sync throughout the body and are what allow us to keep our form and function. Muscles in particular provide the force for movement of body parts, and your muscular system is connected to every other system of the body, including your skeletal system (hence the term *musculoskeletal system*). Muscles play a crucial role in the development of bones and the maintenance of their integrity, and the calcium you absorb with the help of vitamin D in your intestines is also essential for nerve-impulse and muscular functions. Bones are not freewheeling parts. If they weren't attached to your skeletal muscles, with a shared interest in having ample supplies of vitamin D and calcium available, you wouldn't be able to walk, dance, talk, or eat. Your musculoskeletal system is as much part of your survival as is the air you breathe.

So it's no surprise that the intertwining of these two tissues means that what can damage one may also damage the other. Several cross-sectional studies dating years back by Dr. Heike Bischoff-Ferrari and others have shown that a low 25-vitamin D level is related to lower muscle strength, increased body sway, falls, and disability in older men and women. In April of 2000 Dr. Anu Prabhala and his colleagues at SUNY Buffalo reported on the treatment of five patients confined to wheelchairs with severe weakness and fatigue. Blood tests revealed that all suffered from severe vitamin D deficiency. The patients received 50,000 IU of vitamin D per week, and all became mobile within six weeks. Their results were published in *Archives of Internal Medicine*.

Newer evidence further confirms that low levels of vitamin D may be a factor in loss of muscle mass and muscle strength, which we saw at the beginning of this chapter is among the more defining consequences to growing older and weaker. One population-based study from the Netherlands reported that higher levels of circulating 25-vitamin D in both active and sedentary adults sixty years or older were associated with better musculoskeletal function in the legs and lower odds of decline in physical performance as compared to counterparts with lower levels of 25-vitamin D.

Being able to have full function of your legs—not to mention other body parts—later in life can make a significant difference in the ability to stay active and maintain a certain quality of life—which, in turn, affects a person's capacity to continue to maintain and build these lean tissues. Both muscle and bone require the good kind of physical stress that comes with exercise and strength training (weight-bearing exercise) that supports the health of these special tissues. I'll go into more detail about that on page 211.

Recall our two ten-year-old girls from chapter 1 and how, hypothetically speaking, each may face a different fate based on her environment and level of vitamin D. I mentioned that the equatorial girl may be able to jump higher and with more force than her northern counterpart. Why? Because studies have also shown that levels of 25-vitamin D correlate with muscle power and force. One study in particular that was reported in 2009 looked at adolescent girls and revealed that vitamin D is positively related to muscle power, force, velocity, and jump height. This finding alerted researchers to continue investigating this area, because a maturing adolescent with suboptimal muscular force may have long-term consequences in full bone development.

Later in this book, when we get to the how-to's of maintaining optimal levels of vitamin D, I'll elaborate on why physical exercise is so essential to the health and maintenance of your bones and muscles. Adequate vitamin D and calcium intake, along with exercises that stress your musculoskeletal system, constitute the dynamic trio. This is true for both older adults and prepubescent children, whose bone development can be positively influenced by physical activity. Studies continue to come out addressing the perfect storm of not enough vitamin D, not enough calcium, and not enough exercise. Not only does being indoors attached to the computer and television keep children out of the vitamin D–making rays of the sun, but it also keeps them from doing the essential weight-bearing exercises, such as running and jumping, that encourage young bones to grow denser and stronger. What's more, some studies suggest that children and teens today get 20 percent less calcium than is minimally recommended. The culprit? Too much processed food and soda.

Unfortunately, with the recommended daily intake of vitamin D unchanged for over fifty years for children and adults up to fifty years of age, and with our problem of childhood obesity deepening, our youngest generation may be the first generation in the history of humankind to suffer the most health consequences as a result of being deprived of adequate vitamin D. There is no excuse for not getting enough vitamin D when it's freely available from the sun, but we all know that there are plenty of excuses to use in staying out of the sun and forgetting what we're missing. Until it's too late.

CHAPTER 4

Adventures in Globe-Trotting

Do common killers like cancer and heart disease share common geography?

One of the most exciting breakthroughs in my field has been the undeniable connections made between vitamin D deficiency and a higher risk of a variety of cellular health conditions, such as internal cancers, cardiovascular disease, and certain metabolic conditions. Doctors have long understood that sun deprivation causes bone problems, but only relatively recently have these other associations between sunlight and health been made. When epidemiologists (doctors who study the cause and transmission of diseases within populations) ruled out other factors that might explain the better cellular and organ health of people who live in sunnier climates—such as diet, exercise, and alcohol and tobacco use—the search was on to discover the connection between sunshine and decreased risk of certain common diseases.

Those of us in the vitamin D community felt sure there was a connection between this important vitamin and good health. As it turned out, we were right. Increasingly, epidemiologists are discovering that people who live in sunnier climates have a lower incidence of these killer diseases than people who live in climates with are limited amounts of sunlight. Indeed, this is where location means everything.

Location, Location, Location!

Take a look at the following graphics showing cancer rates and blood pressure readings on a map. Find the pattern.

In the next chapter, you'll see a similar pattern when examining the incidence of multiple sclerosis across the map.

As early as the days of World War I it was appreciated that if you lived at a higher latitude, you were at greater risk of dying of cancer—even though it was also appreciated that, yes, if you lived down south and were exposed to more sunlight, you could increase your risk of non-melanoma skin cancer. Following Dr. Peller's analysis of navy personnel, who showed higher rates of nonmelanoma skin cancer but much lower rates of other, more deadly types of cancer than the general public, scientists hunted for further clues to this mysterious connection between

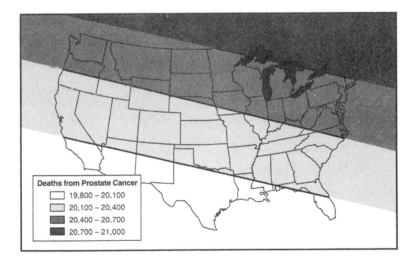

Figure 3. This map shows the rates of prostate cancer in different regions of the United States. As you can tell, the sunnier the region, the fewer prostate deaths there are. The same trend has been identified in analyses of breast and colon cancer rates.

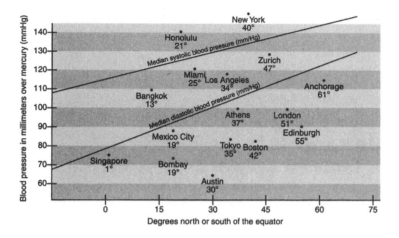

Figure 4. The farther you live from the equator, the higher your blood pressure is likely to be. Why? Because the farther you live from the equator, the less available sun there is to make adequate vitamin D. A New Yorker is likely to have higher blood pressure than someone who lives in Austin, Texas, for example.

how much sun people get throughout the year and their risk of disease. In 1941 Dr. Frank Apperly analyzed cancer statistics throughout North America and Canada. Compared with cities at a latitude between 10 and 30 degrees, cities between 30 and 40 degrees latitude averaged 85 percent higher overall cancer death rates, cities between 40 and 50 degrees latitude averaged 118 percent higher cancer death rates, and cities between 50 and 60 degrees latitude averaged 150 percent higher cancer death rates.

Numerous studies have since confirmed these findings. In the 1980s and 1990s, brothers Cedric and Frank Garland of the University of California at San Diego and Dr. Ed Gorham, among other researchers, picked up where Dr. Apperly had left off and began looking at geography and relating it to cancer incidence. They first looked at colorectal cancer incidence and showed that people living in the northeast had a 10 percent increased risk of developing colorectal cancer. Then they did further studies showing that the higher the latitude at which a person lived, the higher his risk of colorectal, breast, and several other cancers.

Scores of other investigators have found similar associations and further cracked this code of cancer. In 2007, Dr. Joan Lappe and her colleagues at Creighton University reported that postmenopausal women who took 1,400 to 1,500 milligrams of calcium and 1,100 IU of vitamin D daily for four years reduced their risk of developing all cancers by more than 60 percent compared to a placebo group. In my own recent research, after giving mice colon cancer and following them for twenty days, we observed a marked reduction in tumor growth after simply ensuring they got ample vitamin D in their diet. There was a 40 percent reduction in tumor size. This gathering phalanx of research provides strong new evidence that vitamin D could in fact be the single most effective medicine in preventing cancer, perhaps even outpacing the benefits of other preventive measures known to modern science, such as eating a healthy diet.

The bold but unequivocal argument that started with Dr. Peller's and Dr. Apperly's findings continues to gather force today: nonmelanoma skin cancers are relatively easy to detect and treat, unlike lethal colon, prostate, and breast cancer, which we now know are associated with lack of sun exposure. We also know that the sun's protection against cancer is due to vitamin D. You'll have to forgive me for sounding a little repetitive with all this research and published works confirming the same or similar conclusions, the statistics can become dizzying, but they are astonishing. All these insights have truly reshaped our view on sunlight as well as given us a reason to view the last decade as a great leap forward in scientific circles.

Cracking One of Cancer's Codes

A 1990 study published in *Preventive Medicine* showed that women living in the sunnier southwest of the United States were only about half as likely to die from breast cancer as were women in the least sunny northeast region of the country. A 1992 article in the same journal analyzing fifty years of epidemiological cancer data suggested that increasing sun exposure would reduce the number of breast and colon cancer deaths by thirty thousand, or one third.

In 2001, the *Lancet* published an article that directly linked sun exposure to decreased prostate cancer rates. This study showed that British men who had gotten sunburned as children, who vacationed in sunny countries, and who made a habit of sunbathing were much less likely to develop prostate cancer. They also found that people who spent lots of time in the sun tended to develop prostate cancer later than those who spent little time in the sun (at an average of 67.7 years old as compared to 72.1 years). Because prostate cancer grows very slowly, this five-year delay in the age at diagnosis is highly significant.

Two major studies published in 2002 reinforced the link between sunlight and cancer prevention. Doctors from the National Cancer Institute reported that people who either worked outdoors or lived in sunny climates were less likely to die from breast or colon cancer. They also found that the risk of dying from cancers of the ovaries and prostate were lower among people living nearer the equator. In the journal *Cancer* a month earlier, a researcher described how sunlight was responsible for preventing a range of cancers of the reproductive and digestive systems. The study's author, Dr. William Grant, revealed that, compared with residents of the Southwest, people in New England were twice as likely to develop cancers of the breast, ovaries, colon, prostate, bladder, uterus, esophagus, rectum, and stomach.

Based on the statistics available, Grant calculated that in 2002 alone, insufficient sun exposure among Americans caused eighty-five thousand more cases of cancer and thirty thousand more deaths than would have occurred if everyone in the United States had gotten as much sun as people living in the Southwest. Similar observations have been made in Europe.

You may ask, What about the increased rates of melanoma and non-melanoma skin cancer that would, hypothetically, result from this additional sun exposure? Grant calculated the additional number of deaths from skin cancer would be three thousand—a tragically high number, but one far smaller than the number of deaths caused by underexposure to sunlight. Recall that most melanomas occur in the least sun-exposed areas, and working outside in the sun all day (what is sometimes referred to as occupational exposure) lowers one's risk for melanoma. Certain types of cancer have strong gender associations. Breast cancer affects mostly women, and only men get prostate cancer. Both breast and prostate cancer are strongly influenced—in a preventive manner—by sun exposure.

The Garland brothers and their colleagues and Dr. William Grant have shown that if you start out with a 25-vitamin D of at least 20 nanograms per milliliter, you reduce your risk of developing colorectal, breast, and a wide variety of other cancers by 30 percent to 50 percent. It's estimated that if you take 1,000 IU of vitamin D per day, you reduce your risk of developing colorectal, breast, prostate, and ovarian cancer by approximately 50 percent.

Cancer also has strong racial associations. It's well documented that there's a higher incidence of cancer among African Americans than among Caucasians. They also have lower survival rates once diagnosed with cancer. Scientists have long hypothesized that this disparity could be due in part to vitamin D status, as vitamin D deficiency is more prevalent and pronounced among African Americans, whose melanin-rich skin absorbs solar UVB radiation and competes with 7-DHC for these vitamin-D producing rays, thus decreasing the amount of vitamin D that can be manufactured in the skin. When Dr. William Grant reported on this in 2006 for the *Journal of the National Medical Association*, stating that lower cancer survival rates could be attributed to lower 25-vitamin D levels in the black community, he even took factors like smoking, alcohol consumption, access to health care, and poverty into consideration.

Large-scale studies performed by researchers at Harvard found that, after adjusting for multiple dietary, lifestyle, and medical risk factors, African American men were at 32 percent greater risk of total cancer incidence and 89 percent greater risk of total cancer mortality than white men. African American men also have been shown to be at an especially high risk of cancer in the digestive tract (colon, rectum, mouth, esophagus, stomach, and pancreas)—the very group of cancers strongly associated with low 25-vitamin D levels. In 2005, at a meeting of the American Association for Cancer Research, Harvard's lead researcher on these studies, Dr. Edward Giovannucci, a professor of medicine and nutrition, laid out his case in a keynote lecture that had virtually everyone's ears pricked up. His research suggests that vitamin D might help prevent thirty deaths for each one caused by skin cancer.

Breast Cancer

Here's a staggering statistic: Women who are deficient in vitamin D at the time they are diagnosed with breast cancer are nearly 75 percent more likely to die from the disease than women with sufficient vitamin D levels. What's more, their cancer is twice as likely to metastasize to other parts of the body.

In the United States, more than forty thousand women die from breast cancer every year—making it the deadliest killer of women after heart disease. One woman in eight either has or will develop breast cancer in her lifetime. To the more than two hundred thousand women who are diagnosed with this disease each year, there are not only physical consequences but emotional ones too. Self-esteem issues associated with breast cancer can be profound.

There are 214,000 new cases and 41,000 deaths from breast cancer each year in the United States. A 2008 study found that women who had a vitamin D deficiency at the time they were diagnosed with breast cancer were 94 percent more likely to have their cancer spread than women with adequate 25-vitamin D levels in their bodies.

In May 1999, a landmark study by Dr. Esther John, based on the meticulous analysis of breast cancer statistics from the National Health and Nutrition Examination Survey, was published. The results provide extraordinary insight into the relationship between sun exposure and breast cancer. The authors conclude definitively that sun exposure and a vitamin D–rich diet significantly lower the risk of breast cancer.

The John study demonstrates that increased sun exposure alone could potentially reduce the incidence and death rate of breast cancer in the

United States by 35 percent to 75 percent. This would mean that the incidence of new cases might be reduced by 70,000 to 150,000 each year and that 17,500 to 37,500 deaths could be prevented. A conservative estimate is that increased sun exposure could prevent 100,000 new cases of breast cancer and 27,500 deaths from this disease. Combining increased sun exposure with a vitamin D–rich diet or supplements could make the disease prevention and death rate figures 150,000 and 38,000, respectively.

In 2007, researchers pooled the results from two studies—the Harvard Nurses' Health Study and the St. George's Hospital Study in London—and published a report that said patients with the highest blood levels of 25-vitamin D had the lowest risk of breast cancer. Raising 25-vitamin D levels may prevent up to half of breast and two thirds of colorectal cancer cases in the United States alone. In 2008, Dr. Garland and his colleagues again documented an association among a lack of sunlight exposure, low 25-vitamin D, and breast cancer. These statistics likely replicate in other countries at similar latitudes. Based on his studies, Dr. William Grant estimates that lack of sun exposure is responsible for approximately 25 percent of the deaths from breast cancer in Europe. Recently, Dr. Julia Knight of the University of Toronto reported that women who had the most sun exposure as teenagers and young adults had a more than 60 percent reduced risk of developing breast cancer compared to women who had the least sun exposure. One can only imagine the excitement that would result if a drug were invented that yielded such preventive results!

Again, you might ask about skin cancer rates. Wouldn't they rise in response to increased sun exposure? Approximately 500 women a year die from nonmelanoma skin cancer. Given that the above statistics show that 27,500 women die prematurely because of underexposure to sunlight, it becomes evident that 55 women die prematurely because of underexposure to sunlight for every 1 who dies prematurely from overexposure to sunlight.

Hang tight: I'll be answering all your questions about sunlight and skin cancer in chapter 8. For now, let's keep the focus on the types of cancer that kill more people and don't cry mercy too often when diagnosed and treated.

Prostate Cancer

Only heart attacks and lung cancer kill more men than cancer of the prostate, which every year claims more than fifty thousand lives in the United States alone. Prostate cancer kills one in four men who get this disease, making it one of the most deadly forms of cancer. About forty thousand American men die every year from prostate cancer—more than ten times as many as are killed by melanomas.

Cancer of the prostate is especially feared by men because surgical treatment for this form of cancer frequently results in impotence. A study in the August 2001 issue of the *Lancet* proves that the risk of developing prostate cancer is directly related to sunlight exposure. The study divided people into four groups according to how much sunlight they had been exposed to. The lowest quarter, or quartile, of the study participants were three times more likely to develop prostate cancer than those in the highest quartile of sun exposure. The results show that those in the highest quartile reduced their risk of developing prostate cancer by 66 percent. Those in the second and third quartiles also had a significantly lower chance of getting prostate cancer compared with those in the lowest quartile, who received the least sun exposure. Another study took a long look, over almost two years, at men with prostate cancer who received 2,000 IU of vitamin D a day and found that overall the men had a 50 percent reduction in the rise of their levels of prostate-specific antigen (PSA), which is an indicator of prostate cancer activity.

Only about six hundred men die prematurely each year from nonmelanoma skin cancer, but thirty-seven thousand men die prematurely each year from prostate cancer. It's possible to conclude that fifty-five men die prematurely from underexposure to sunlight for every one who dies prematurely due to overexposure. Even when you include melanoma—for which excessive sunshine is only one of several risk factors—the numbers are still lopsided: about ten to one.

Colon Cancer

Cancer of the colon and its neighboring area, known sometimes as colorectal cancer, affects both men and women. Like breast cancer and prostate cancer, colorectal cancer is seen much more frequently than skin cancers and is much more deadly. About 150,000 Americans are told each year that they have colon cancer, and about 35 percent of these will die of it. There are many contributing factors in why someone gets colon cancer, but the most commonly acknowledged one is diet. Diets high in fat and nonorganic non-grass-fed red meat are especially dangerous. Other diets, such as diets high in fruits, vegetables, and other natural raw and organic foods, help prevent colon cancer.

A study published in the *Journal of Clinical Oncology* in 2008, conducted by lead researcher Dr. Kimmie Ng of the Dana-Farber Cancer Institute in Boston found that high blood levels of 25 vitamin D increased colon cancer patients' survival rate by 48 percent. In this study, Dr. Ng and her team collected data on 304 patients who had been diagnosed with colon cancer between 1991 and 2002. Everyone in the study had had their 25-vitamin D blood levels measured a minimum of two years before being diagnosed with the disease. The patients were tracked until they died or until the study ended in 2005; 123 patients died, 96 of them from colon or rectal cancer during the follow-up period. Dr. Ng and her team found that the patients with the highest 25-vitamin D levels were 39 percent less likely to die from colorectal cancer than the patients who had the lowest levels.

These findings are consistent with dozens and dozens of other observations that have been made in the past decade, including those by Dr. Cedric Garland. His lab reports that you are three times less likely to die from colon cancer if you have healthy levels of 25-vitamin D in your bloodstream.

How Vitamin D Takes the Life out of Cancer

The link between vitamin D and cancer may have gained a strong foothold just recently within the medical community at large, but the research started long ago. Toward the end of the 1980s, I was part of a small but growing movement of medical scientists who believed that the active form of vitamin D that I had discovered a decade earlier had benefits well beyond bone health. We theorized that people who lived in sunnier climates had lower rates of cancer and heart disease because the vitamin D produced by their exposure to the sun was somehow benefiting cells throughout the body. A few studies backed this up at the time, but what exactly was causing this?

My fellow researchers had successfully proved the relationship between sunlight and cellular health, but I believed their conclusion as to why sunlight and increased vitamin D production benefited cellular health was incorrect. They thought that vitamin D benefited cells throughout the body in the same way we understood it benefited bone health. That is, the more sunshine you get, the more 25-vitamin D there is circulating in your bloodstream that can be converted by the kidneys into activated vitamin D. According to this theory, this activated vitamin D would then be sent by the kidneys to different parts of the body, where it would benefit different cell groups by regulating their growth and preventing them from becoming malignant. This theory assumes that the more vitamin D you get from the sun and your diet, the more activated vitamin D your kidneys will make.

I believed something quite different. At the time, my theory was considered heretical, and it probably still would be if my colleagues and I hadn't proved it. We understood that activated vitamin D is one of the most potent inhibitors of abnormal cell growth, but we knew that no matter how much you increased the supply of 25-vitamin D in a person's body through sunlight and diet, you couldn't get the kidneys to make any additional activated vitamin D. I didn't think the very limited amount of activated vitamin D the kidneys are able to produce could be responsible for all the cellular benefits that we had identified. In other words, the kidneys could not be the sole ruler in the vitamin D land. I believed that there had to be another source of activated vitamin D.

What my colleagues and I proposed was that cells throughout the body don't have to rely on the meager supply of activated vitamin D from the kidneys because each group of cells has its own enzymatic machinery to convert 25-vitamin D into activated vitamin D. In other words, cells can make their own activated vitamin D on the spot without having to rely on activated vitamin D sent from the distant kidneys. (If this story sounds familiar, that's because I told it earlier from a slightly different angle and in broader strokes.)

We proved this theory in a study published in 1998 that involved collaboration with Dr. Gary Schwartz and my colleague Dr. Tai Chen. Our findings completely changed the way medical science perceives the relationship between vitamin D and cellular and organ health. In this study we exposed normal prostate cells to 25-vitamin D to see what would happen. The cells converted 25-vitamin D to activated vitamin D (1,25-vitamin D). We then exposed prostate cancer cells to 25-vitamin D. In cancerous fashion, these cells were reproducing out of control. When we exposed these prostate cancer cells to 25-vitamin D, they converted that substance into activated vitamin D and stopped their chaotic reproduction. What we had actually proved was that, just like the kidney, normal prostate cells and prostate cancer cells could make activated vitamin D. But unlike the activated vitamin D made by the kidneys, which regulates calcium metabolism and promotes bone health, the activated vitamin D created within the prostate has the job of ensuring healthy cell growth. Not only was this confirmed in subsequent studies, but similar studies by my research group and other researchers found that the same enzymatic machinery to activate vitamin D also exists in the cells of the colon, breast, lung, and brain.

This finding helped make more sense out of other mysteries about the body's use of vitamin D. The vitamin D activated in the kidneys specifically travels to the intestine and bone to regulate calcium metabolism. So if your kidneys were to make a lot more active vitamin D, there would be negative health consequences, such as hypercalcemia (high blood calcium) and hypercalciuria (high urine calcium). What the body cleverly does instead is allow other tissues and cells in your body to activate vitamin D. If you have a patient who has no kidneys, he has no circulating blood levels of activated vitamin D. Therefore, it used to be assumed that only the kidneys made activated vitamin D. What was shown by my lab and others was that the body was smarter and could activate vitamin D locally in the prostate, colon, and breast.

Activated vitamin D, locally produced, can regulate up to two thousand different genes that control cell growth and other cellular functions, produce insulin in the pancreas, and regulate production of the hormone renin in the kidneys. Once it carries out these functions, activated vitamin D triggers the expression of 25-vitamin D-24-hydroxylase, which is an enzyme that rapidly destroys activated vitamin D. Activated vitamin D never leaves the cell, and therefore its signature is never picked up in the bloodstream. It's a silent soldier that essentially commits suicide once its task is finished on site. Another brilliant example of how the body self-regulates.

The consequences of this discovery are mind-boggling. We had discovered the likely reason why sun exposure has such a profound effect on cancer rates. When you are exposed to more sunlight and make more vitamin D, it can be converted by the liver into 25-vitamin D, which can be activated by the prostate, colon, ovaries, breast, pancreas, brain, and probably most other tissues to prevent unhealthy cell growth. The more 25-vitamin D you make, the healthier these disease-prone tissues will be. Because we don't have to rely on a supply of activated vitamin D from our kidneys, there is an enormous capacity to prevent cancer just by having ample supplies of 25-vitamin D around that originate either from the sunlight's action in the skin or from supplementation of vitamin D_2 or D_3. Powerful new synthetic forms of activated vitamin D also are being studied to see how they could hinder cancer growth.

While the potential for activated vitamin D to be used as a treatment for cancer seems logical given vitamin D's preventive actions on cells, there's more to the cancer story that bears understanding. For one thing, cancer cells are clever. Once a malignancy takes hold, those cancerous cells begin to make more of a protein that controls the expression of genes, called a transcription factor. And one of those transcription factors, called Snail, binds to the vitamin D receptor and renders it dysfunctional. Once that happens, activated vitamin D can no longer regulate gene expression and thus can no longer work on cells to protect them. It's like a switch that's been flipped off. The cancerous cells essentially become closed for business with activated vitamin D and, left to their own devices, continue to grow and inflict harm on nearby tissues.

A New Model for Cancer?

Though it's a stretch to say vitamin D can totally prevent and cure cancer, some scientists have been bold enough to suggest a whole new theory about cancer.

Just last year, the Garland brothers raised the possibility that there's another story behind cancer's genesis in the body. The current scientific model assumes that a genetic mutation is cancer's point of origin. But what if that assumption is wrong? What if there is another way to explain how cancer develops? Those are the questions the Garlands put forth, which were published in the *Annals of Epidemiology* and immediately picked up by the media.

First, Dr. Cedric Garland and his team pointed to a host of research that suggests cancer develops when cells lose the ability to stick together in a healthy, normal way. He went on to argue that the key factor in this initial triggering of a malignancy could well be a lack of vitamin D. According to Dr. Garland, researchers have documented that with enough activated vitamin D present, cells adhere to one another in tissue and act as normal, mature cells. But if there is a deficiency of activated vitamin D, cells can lose this stick-to-each-other quality, as well as their identity as differentiated cells. The result? They may revert to a dangerous, immature state and become cancerous.

What can stop this process from occurring, says Dr. Garland, is ample supplies of vitamin D in the body. When enough activated vitamin D is present, it may halt the first stage of the cancer process by reestablishing connections among cells that have an intact vitamin D receptor. No activated vitamin D around, no action on the cell to help change its course.

This new model of cancer's cause has been dubbed DINOMIT by Dr. Garland and his colleagues. Each letter stands for a different phase of cancer development: *D* refers to disjunction, or loss of communication between cells; *I* is for initiation, when genetic mutations begin to play a role; *N* refers to natural selection of the fastest-reproducing cancer cells; *O* is for overgrowth of cells; *M* stands for metastasis, the spread of a malignancy to other tissues; *I* refers to involution and *T* for transition, both dormant states that may occur in cancer and can potentially be altered by increasing vitamin D.

Whether or not this theory can be proven true will be told by future studies and research. Clues about a possible cause-and-effect association between a lack of vitamin D and cancer's development have rapidly accumulated over the past few years. No doubt more clues will continue to mount and slowly crush the incessant chatter that sunlight is always bad and that skin cancer should be first and foremost on everyone's worry list.

I could go on and on listing studies; theories associating vitamin D with many cancers have been tested and confirmed in over two hundred epidemiological studies. In addition, more than 2,500 laboratory studies have been conducted that provide an understanding of the physiological basis of vitamin D's link to cancer. See for yourself: Google *vitamin D and cancer* and you'll find thousands of links to papers and articles pouring out of the most prestigious universities and research centers around the world. The flip side of this optimistic coin, though, is the fact that most cancer patients are vitamin D deficient. My own studies, in addition to others, have documented this, and it is not a surprise given that the general population's level of 25-vitamin D is, for the most part, woefully deficient. Add to that the fact that cancer patients usually don't feel well, so they're not outside and are not active, and often have upset stomachs, so they are not eating very well and as a result are not fully absorbing whatever little vitamin D may be in their diet. My team has found that when we give cancer patients vitamin D, they report feeling better. Their muscle strength improves, and their overall feeling of well-being climbs.

Beating Down Heart Disease

When you look back at the graph on page 76 that shows blood pressure rates across different latitudes, you'll see that the farther away from the equator you live, the higher your blood pressure gets. What gives? Is it in the air? The water? The food? No, it's in the sky—the sun, or lack thereof.

Because of vitamin D's actions in the body, sun exposure has a dramatic effect on heart and circulatory disease. High blood pressure, also known as hypertension, is a very serious condition that is the main cause of stroke and heart attack. If you live in a sunny climate, you are less likely to have high blood pressure than if you live somewhere with less sunlight at certain times of the year. People tend to have healthier blood pressure during the summer than during the winter because there's more sunlight available—and thus more vitamin D in the body. When exposed to the same amount of sunlight, people with fairer skin have healthier blood pressure than those with dark skin, thanks to higher levels of vitamin D (the darker your skin, the more melanin there is in it, and consequently the more difficult it is for you to produce vitamin D from the sun). There's now specific evidence that people who live in sunnier climates have fewer heart attacks. Heart failure is also associated with vitamin D deficiency.

The Heart of the Matter

Scientists now believe that the work we did on the mechanism of action of activated vitamin D on cell growth also has a bearing on those cells important to heart and circulatory health, especially the blood vessels. Blood vessels are the tubular channels—the arteries and veins—through which blood circulates throughout your body. High blood pressure can occur if the blood vessels get stiff and narrow, which increases the pressure inside them.

The work showing that there are vitamin D receptors in various cells throughout the body and that these cells activate vitamin D led me and other scientists to conclude that there are also vitamin D receptors in the cells of our blood vessels. The effect of vitamin D on the blood vessels is to make them relax and be more flexible. It does this in two ways. It lessens the effects on the blood vessels of the renin-angiotensin system, which is a complex hormone system that regulates blood pressure and water balance in the body, and it works directly on vessels and smooth muscle to relax them. Thus, the blood flows more efficiently through them, because there is less pressure against the blood vessel walls. What's more, when 25-vitamin D levels are low, calcium can accumulate in artery walls and promote formation of dangerous fatty plaques. And it's the breakup of these plaques that leads to the occlusions and clots that are the direct causes of heart attacks, heart failure, and strokes.

At the same time, bones can be deprived of calcium as vitamin D deficiency prevents proper absorption of calcium from the intestines. This constitutes a double whammy: weaker bones and sick arteries, as calcium accumulates in the wrong area. This hardening of the arteries is also known as atherosclerosis.

Women with osteoporosis tend to have more calcium in the walls of their arteries, and they run a greater risk of cardiac death than women with strong, dense bones.

Research into the link between low 25-vitamin D and cardiovascular trouble dates back twenty years. In 1990, Professor Robert Scragg of the University of Auckland published the discovery that heart attack victims had lower 25-vitamin D levels than their healthy counterparts. His team examined two sets of blood samples, one taken from 179 heart-attack patients within twelve hours of the onset of symptoms, and another taken from healthy people on the same day. This control group matched the heart patients in terms of age and gender distribution. Dr. Scragg's group found that the heart-attack patients had a significantly lower average 25-vitamin D level than the healthy controls. The risk of a heart attack was calculated as being 57 percent lower among the people with higher 25-vitamin D levels than among those with lower levels.

In 2002, more evidence emerged when a team of researchers led by Dr. Paul Varosy at the University of California at San Francisco looked at nearly ten thousand women over age sixty-five who had participated in an earlier study of osteoporotic fractures. Some of these women either had taken supplemental vitamin D in the past or were continuing to do so. Dr. Varosy was hoping to find out how taking a supplement would impact the women's risk for heart-related problems. After following the women for an average of about eleven years, he determined that those who used vitamin D supplements enjoyed a 31 percent reduction in the risk of heart disease–related death compared with women who did not. The researchers were quick to point out that the use of calcium supplements did not affect their results. They also managed to weed out other factors that potentially could have skewed their results, including diet, genetics, lifestyle, health conditions, and education.

I have participated in several studies over the last two decades to investigate the effects of UVB irradiation on heart health. Dr. Rolfdeiter Krause and my colleagues and I have found that regularly exposing patients with high blood pressure to UVB radiation in a tanning bed caused their blood pressure to become normal—in other words, they got healthier. The best known of these studies was published in the *Lancet* back in 1998. In this study, we showed that exposing hypertensive patients to brief periods of UVB radiation in a tanning bed three times a week for three months elevated bloodstream 25-vitamin D by 180 percent and reduced diastolic blood pressure by 6 millimeters of mercury (mmHg) and systolic blood pressure by 6 mmHg, bringing them into the normal range. (That's about as much as most blood-pressure medications do, but without the unpleasant side effects!)

How did we know that the UVB radiation was at work rather than the warmth and relaxing environment effecting this change? We provided the same treatments to a separate set of hypertensive patients using a UVA tanning bed, and this made no difference to 25-vitamin D levels or blood pressure. For the entire nine months we followed them, those patients who continued with the tanning-bed treatments maintained a healthier, lower blood pressure. Remember that high blood pressure is one of the leading causes of death in the United States and the rest of the industrialized world because it is a main cause of heart attack and stroke and a major cause of kidney failure.

My colleagues and I also studied areas of heart health other than hypertension. I was part of a team of researchers who, to confirm the pioneering work of Drs. Malte Bühring and Rolfdeiter Krause, exposed a group of heart-disease patients to UVB radiation three times a week for a month. Increasing 25-vitamin D levels in the body in this way improved heart health in a variety of ways—heart strength (as measured by blood-pumping ability) was increased and heart strain (as measured by resting and nonresting heart rate and the accumulation of lactic acid) was decreased. Our studies and other research teams' efforts show that the benefits of UVB to heart health are similar to those of an exercise program. And, as I mentioned earlier, when combined with physical fitness, UVB exposure has been shown to have extremely beneficial results.

If you take people with hypertension and put them in a tanning bed for brief periods that simulates sunlight three times a week for three months, you can increase their blood level of 25-vitamin D by as much as 180 percent and lower their blood pressure to normal levels—no drugs required.

In 2006, an Italian team of researchers measured the amount of atherosclerotic plaque in the arteries of 390 diabetic patients, as well as the patients' 25-vitamin D levels. What did they find? Low 25-vitamin D blood levels were associated strongly with a greater degree of atherosclerosis. Later that year, the same team found vitamin D deficiencies in three out of five people diagnosed with type 2 diabetes. The rate of vitamin D deficiency was 61 percent in the diabetics versus only 43 percent in the nondiabetic controls. This was in line with the team's previous finding, as the 31 percent of the diabetics with cardiovascular disease were very likely to also have low blood levels of 25-vitamin D.

Most recently, a study led by Dr. Thomas Wang at Harvard Medical School and published in the American Heart Association's journal, *Circulation*, unveiled astounding statistics regarding the relationship of vitamin D deficiency to one's risk of heart attacks, strokes, and other cardiovascular events. Researchers followed 1,739 people for five years, assessing their 25-vitamin D levels by means of regular blood tests. The average age of participants was fifty-nine. All participants were white, had no prior history of cardiovascular disease, and were the children of the original participants in a landmark, multigenerational study called the Framingham Heart Study.

Participants with low levels of 25-vitamin D had a 60 percent higher chance of experiencing a cardiovascular event, including heart attack, heart failure, or stroke, during the study period than participants with high blood levels. Another study has further showed that people who in fact do suffer heart attacks are more likely to survive it if they are vitamin D sufficient as opposed to insufficient or deficient. (Note that this pretty much confirms exactly what Dr. Scragg observed twenty years ago.) The correlation remained even after researchers adjusted for other risk factors such as diabetes, high blood pressure, and high cholesterol. Those who had both vitamin D deficiency and high blood pressure had *twice* the risk of cardiovascular events as those who had vitamin D deficiency alone. The results of the studies treating heart and circulatory health with UVB radiation demonstrate why people who spend time in the sun tend to have healthier blood pressure and better all-around heart health.

At the American Headache Society's fiftieth annual meeting in 2008, vitamin D got a round of applause when Dr. Steve Wheeler from the Ryan Wheeler Headache Treatment Center in Miami presented his story. Turns out he had been reading up on vitamin D deficiency in the medical literature, coming across several of my studies, and this prompted him to take a look at the vitamin D status of his patients suffering from chronic migraine. Migraines are unique types of headaches that typically entail throbbing, pulsating pain on one side of the head, accompanied by nausea and sensitivity to light. To a large extent, migraines remain a mystery, but we know they are related to blood-vessel contractions and other changes in the brain. Dr. Wheeler noticed that no one had ever looked at the vitamin D status of the forty-five million migraineurs, yet patients with migraine often have other health concerns such as increased risk for cardiovascular disease, cerebro-vascular disease, and fibromyalgia—all conditions that have also been linked to vitamin D deficiency.

But first, Dr. Wheeler started with himself. A migraine sufferer, he discovered that his 25-vitamin D levels were drastically low, a scanty 8.2 nanograms per milliliter. Dr. Wheeler was inspired to immediately start testing his patients, finding that 41.8 percent of the fifty-five patients he assessed at a single outpatient laboratory over a six-month period had sub-optimal levels of vitamin D. Specifically, 27.3 percent of these 41.8 percent of people had insufficient levels (between 20 and 30 nanograms per milliliter) and 14.5 percent had deficient levels (20 nanograms per milliliter or below).

Dr. Wheeler's examination confirmed what other studies had previously found. There was a trend toward hypertension and type 2 diabetes in his vitamin D–deficient patients. His team also uncovered a trend toward earlier onset of headache (14.3 years of age versus 18) and migraine (16.7 years old versus 22.2) in his vitamin D–deficient patients. Those with vitamin D insufficiency were more likely to have osteopenia (the precursor to osteoporosis), and those deficient were more likely to have osteoporosis. This prompted Dr. Wheeler to conclude that vitamin D deficiency is an unrecognized yet treatable cause of cardiovascular disease and could aggravate problems with migraine.

The Beat Goes On

Finally, there's one more study I want to point out related to the cardiovascular system that just came out in 2009, this one from Sweden. Forty thousand women had been followed for about eleven years, one thousand women per year of age from twenty-five to sixty-four. The goal of the study was to see if sun-exposure habits were related to the risk of so-called venous thromboembolism (VTE) events, which, in simple terms, are blood clots in the veins. These can be deadly. About six hundred thousand Americans develop VTE each year, and one hundred thousand of those die. VTE includes deep vein thrombosis (DVT), in which clots form in the deep veins, often in the legs, and when let loose travel to the lungs, causing a pulmonary embolism.

Swedish women who sunbathed during the summer, on winter vacations, or when abroad or used a tanning bed were at 30 percent lower risk of VTE than those who did not. This percentage did not change even after the scientists made adjustments for demographic variables. The risk of VTE increased by 50 percent in winter as compared to the other seasons. And, not too surprisingly, the lowest risk was found in the summer. The researchers speculated that greater UVB radiation exposure was the reason. It improves levels of vitamin D, which in turn enhances the body's anticoagulant (declotting) properties and improves conditions in the body that help prevent such catastrophic clots.

Hypertension: The Silent Killer

One in four adult Americans—fifty million in all—suffers from hypertension, the main sign of which is high blood pressure. More than half of Americans (67 percent) older than sixty have hypertension. It's expected to affect 1.6 billion people worldwide by the year 2025. Despite its prevalence, high blood pressure is often ignored or undiagnosed because it has no symptoms. However, hypertension is a prime risk factor for heart disease and stroke, the first and third leading causes of death in this country. It's a chief factor in our nation's struggle with chronic disease, disability, and even death. Because it is an insidious and deadly disease, hypertension is sometimes called the silent killer.

We know that blood vessels have vitamin D receptors. The active form of vitamin D will enhance contraction of the heart muscle and improve vascular smooth-muscle function, as Dr. Robert U. Simpson from the University of Michigan showed many years ago. We know that activated vitamin D alters inflammatory activity, which is a major factor in the development of atherosclerosis. And there is evidence that the active form of vitamin D regulates the major blood-pressure-regulating hormone renin in your kidneys. The gathering evidence on vitamin D's active role in regulating blood pressure has prompted numerous studies lately, as researchers continue to look for clues to conquering this silent killer.

Blood Sugar and Metabolic Syndrome

High blood pressure. High blood sugar. Unhealthy cholesterol and triglyceride levels. Excess abdominal (belly) fat. If you were to look into a crowd of Americans, say, at a football game or large concert, and start counting how many of them could check off all of these conditions as relating to them, you'd be tagging one of every six people. That's forty-seven million Americans. Collectively, this set of conditions has a strange name: metabolic syndrome, or, stranger still, syndrome X. You may not intuitively put high blood pressure, for example, in the same category as metabolism, but all of these conditions share a unique relationship. And when they combine in the body, they can have an epic impact. These risk factors double your risk of blood-vessel and heart disease, which can lead to heart attacks and strokes. They increase your risk of diabetes by five times.

When you hear the word *diabetes*, most likely it's related to type 2, so-called adult onset diabetes. It's the most common form of diabetes; of the 23.6 million people with diabetes, 90 percent to 95 percent have type 2. Like type 1, this form disrupts the body's ability to metabolize sugar for fuel, but type 2 is not an autoimmune disease. In type 2 diabetes, the beta cells of the pancreas continue to make insulin, but when there is too much fat, there is a resistance to insulin, so the body cannot use it effectively. When that happens, a person is said to be insulin resistant and prediabetic. As the disease progresses, insulin production slows down after several years, and the result is similar to what occurs in type 1 diabetes: glucose, the body's preferred form of energy, builds up in the blood and the body cannot make efficient use of its main source of fuel.

Unlike type 1, which I'll describe in the next chapter as being autoimmune related, this form of diabetes is associated with older age, obesity, a family history of diabetes, physical inactivity, and ethnicity. About 80 percent of people with type 2 diabetes are overweight, which is why this type gets so much media exposure now that obesity rates have soared. For some, reversing this disease is possible through changes in diet and exercise habits. But for others, the ravages of this disease can make for a long struggle that destroys the quality of life and brings a complicated morass of medical challenges.

Because activated vitamin D can increase insulin production, it's no surprise that research has indicated that UVB radiation—and hence, adequate levels of 25-vitamin D in the body—may have an indirect role in preventing type 2 diabetes. We have yet to learn the exact effect vitamin D has on the risk for type 2 diabetes, but the evidence continues to collect showing a clear association between sufficient vitamin D and efficient cellular metabolism. Numerous longitudinal studies have consistently demonstrated that people who suffer from type 2 diabetes typically have low 25-vitamin D levels. Just last year a team of scientists from Harvard and Tufts reported in the *Journal of Nutrition* that vitamin D status may be an important determinant for type 2 diabetes, based on their findings when studying the relationship between 25-vitamin D levels and insulin resistance.

What we do know is that a lack of vitamin D is related to both insulin resistance and impaired pancreatic beta cells, which are the sources of insulin for the body's metabolism and which do possess vitamin D receptors. In studies done with mice, beta cells lose their capacity to secrete insulin when their vitamin D receptor isn't functioning as it should because of low 25-vitamin D.

In 2004, researchers at UCLA unveiled their findings after trying to make better sense of the CARDIA (Coronary Artery Risk Development in Young Adults) Study, a population-based look at vitamin D's role in metabolic syndrome. The CARDIA Study examined a sampling of 3,157 black and white adults aged eighteen to thirty years from four metropolitan areas in the United States. What it found was that among overweight adults, the more milk people drank, the less likely they were to be insulin resistant. The numbers, in fact, are quite staggering—people with the highest dairy consumption had a 72 percent lower incidence of metabolic syndrome. The study concluded that dairy consumption could reduce the risk of type 2 diabetes and cardiovascular disease. The UCLA team confirmed this conclusion in its own study and reported specifically on how higher levels of 25-vitamin D correlated to this lowered risk.

Even more revealing have been the studies done on the effect both vitamin D and calcium—the high-powered couple we'll explore again in chapter 9—can have on reducing one's risk for diabetes. One large study published in 2006 by *Diabetes Care* that looked at middle-aged women concluded that a high daily intake of vitamin D (greater than 800 IU) and calcium (greater than 1,200 milligrams) was associated with a 33 percent lower risk of type 2 diabetes.

Type 2 diabetics tend to be stuck in a vicious cycle whereby they battle weight problems and lack the energy or motivation to exercise, precipitating other health challenges—from their overworked organs to their inability to get a good night's sleep. The number of potential hazards that flow from their condition and resulting secondary conditions is practically limitless. Add to that a vitamin D deficiency, knowing all the areas in which vitamin D can have a positive impact, and you can quickly grasp the magnitude and intricacy of this problem. Achieving a break in the cycle typically requires a complete lifestyle and dietary change, as well as a focus on reducing stress levels that can thwart weight-loss efforts and perpetuate hormonal imbalances.

In the last few years, the spotlight has been turned on teens, who are currently changing the actuarial tables. Soaring obesity rates among our adolescents may actually shift their longevity, snipping two to five years off their life spans as compared to their parents'. And new research has also linked low levels of 25-vitamin D to high blood pressure and high blood sugar in this age group—the very risk factors for heart disease and conditions associated with this elusive metabolic syndrome. A team of researchers led by Jared Reis of Johns Hopkins's Bloomberg School of Public Health found that teens (3,600 boys and girls ages twelve to nineteen) with the lowest 25-vitamin D levels were more than twice as likely to have high blood pressure and high blood sugar than those with higher 25-vitamin D levels. They were also four times more likely to have metabolic syndrome than their counterparts with optimal levels of 25-vitamin D. The vitamin D–deficiency pattern was consistent with earlier findings in that blacks had the lowest levels, followed by the Mexican Americans; whites had the highest levels, but all of the teens showed a deficiency. Further research will determine the extent to which vitamin D lies behind these health problems and how much of an impact it can have in preventing, treating, and reversing these problems.

Do you have a teenager who is vitamin D deficient? New research proves teens with low levels of vitamin D have a high risk of high blood pressure and blood sugar, which can contribute to heart disease and other serious conditions.

CHAPTER 5

Finding Immunity

Can vitamin D be the body's secret weapon against germs and autoimmune disease?

I n addition to responding to the *New York Times* or CNN, some of my proudest moments have been responding to feedback after landing in such esteemed publications as *People*, the *National Enquirer,* and the *Globe* (not the *Boston Globe*, but rather the tabloid you find at supermarket checkouts).

In the late 1980s I went to a dermatology meeting and gave a talk on a Friday afternoon about my clinical research using activated vitamin D to treat psoriasis. This was just after I had tried to publish a study on activated vitamin D's profound effects on this painful skin disorder when applied topically in an ointment. The *New England Journal of Medicine* had flatly rejected my submission. But that didn't mean I couldn't go and report my findings to local dermatologists, hoping a few inquisitive souls would listen.

As you can imagine, there weren't many people present at that time of day on the eve of a weekend. Half a roomful of people showed up, looking eager to end the workweek. I was told, though, that the *Boston Globe* was there fishing for a human-interest story. I presented my results and recommended this new treatment for psoriasis. I had shown in clinical trials that adding active vitamin D to Vaseline and applying it topically could dramatically reduce the excessive cell proliferation that causes psoriasis. Well, suffice it to say my talk ultimately wound up being picked up in the other "Globe" publication (the second-most-read tabloid in the world) several months later under the headline "Break-through for Psoriasis: Call Holick" (strategically placed right next to news about then-popular primetime soap *Dynasty*).

My phone was ringing off the hook the following week. More than twenty thousand people suffering from psoriasis wrote to me asking to participate in my study.

Today, my method has become one of the first-line treatments for psoriasis. I had one of the largest psoriasis patient populations of any dermatologist in the country and continue to treat psoriasis patients with activated forms of vitamin D.

The Betrayal

It may seen unfathomable that the body could turn against itself and inflict harm by ordering the immune system to attack its own tissues and cells. But that's exactly what happens in the case of autoimmune diseases such as multiple sclerosis, type 1 diabetes, and rheumatoid arthritis. These can be among the most perplexing illnesses or conditions to study and try to understand from a purely scientific and evolutionary standpoint. How can Mother Nature let this happen? How many triggers of autoimmune diseases are there? Will we ever find the silver bullet to reset an immune system gone awry?

Psoriasis, while typically placed under the "autoimmune diseases" umbrella, is not actually an autoimmune disease. I'll explain why I don't like calling it an autoimmune disease a bit later in this chapter. Psoriasis deserves attention alongside the more official autoimmune illnesses, though, because it involves the immune system at some point in its progression. Controversy continues to swirl around psoriasis's story, but you'll find that to be the case for most of the mysterious autoimmune diseases that have yet to be fully decoded and categorized as bona fide autoimmune diseases or something else entirely. One thing is certain: psoriasis is probably one of the longest-known illnesses of humans and simultaneously one of the most misunderstood. Similarly, vitamin D may be the oldest hormone on the planet and one of the most misunderstood. The odd couple indeed.

Your Automatic Weapon

Surely you have some memory from high-school biology about the immune system—the intricate system of special cells that defend the body against invading microorganisms, such as viruses and bacteria. The immune system does this by producing antibodies or particular kinds of white blood cells, called sensitized lymphocytes, to attack these unwelcome invaders.

If your immune system is working as it should, it won't attack fellow cells; it will only respond to threats from real trespassers. But if something goes wrong, your immune system can malfunction and signal antibodies and sensitized lymphocytes to attack your own cells. This usually occurs because of an external disturbance of your immune system by a medication, bacteria, or virus, combined with a genetic predisposition to autoimmune disease. While it may be ironic that the body can become a victim of its own design, as the very system set up to deal with invaders can be tricked by them, a gathering body of evidence implicates outsiders as the instigators of a wide variety of autoimmune diseases. The immune system, it turns out, may not be as infallible as we'd like. But that makes the case for its connection to vitamin D all the stronger.

As was recently discovered, one of the main reasons for this disproportionate incidence of autoimmune diseases across the globe may be the vitamin D receptors of the immune system. Because immune cells have vitamin D receptors (VDRs), they may benefit from the vitamin D the body generates from sun exposure. After all, why would these cells have receptors for vitamin D if there weren't a purpose for them and a concomitant need for vitamin D to act on them?

And, as we explored previously, vitamin D also promotes other areas of cellular health, which makes it less likely that an undesirable autoimmune response will occur. In other words, when the body is functioning optimally and has all the ingredients it needs to fulfill its cellular obligations, conditions are ideal and there's less likely to be a mishap somewhere in the millions of reactions that take place every day without your even thinking about them. Because of the mounting evidence that sun exposure is an effective preventive measure against autoimmune diseases, activated vitamin D and artificial forms of this substance (known as activated vitamin D analogs) are increasingly being tested as a therapy for diseases that have an autoimmune component.

Sickness Where the Sun Doesn't Shine So Bright

For some time, epidemiologists have known that autoimmune diseases are less common in regions close to the equator, where there is more sunshine throughout the year. The following graphic should look a little similar to the ones in the last chapter.

The connection between sun exposure and multiple sclerosis (MS), for example, is undisputed. The disease is about five times more likely to affect you if you live in North America or Europe than if you live

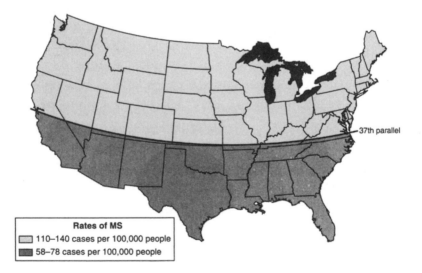

Figure 5. Similar to the pattern of cancer and blood pressure rates across the country, the higher the latitude, the higher the rates of multiple sclerosis. A jump in MS cases are reported among those who live above the 37th parallel. It has been reported that if you live above the 37th parallel for the first ten years of your life, you have 100 percent increased risk of developing MS for the rest of your life, no matter where you live.

in the tropics. In the United States, MS is far more prevalent in states above the 37th parallel than in states below it. From east to west, the 37th parallel extends from Newport News, Virginia, to Santa Cruz, California, and runs along the northern border of North Carolina and west to the northern border of Arizona and across California. The MS prevalence rates for the region below the 37th parallel are 57 to 78 cases per 100,000 people. The prevalence rates for the region above the 37th parallel are almost double that: 110 to 140 cases per 100,000 people.

Multiple sclerosis is a chronic, debilitating disease that affects the brain and spinal cord, which together make up the central nervous system. In MS, the body sends immune cells to the brain and spinal cord, resulting in nerve damage to these structures. Eventually, multiple areas of scarring (sclerosis) develop, causing slowed or blocked muscle coordination, weakness, double vision, and eventually loss of sight and other nerve signals. Most people develop MS between the ages of twenty and forty. An estimated 400,000 Americans have MS, and there are thought to be 2.5 million sufferers worldwide. The disease is at least twice as common in women as in men.

There is a well-established genetic component in MS—if someone in your family had the disease, you are much more likely to get it. About 20 percent of people with MS have at least one affected relative. If you're a first-degree relative, such as a child or a sibling, of someone with MS, your chance of eventually developing MS is twenty to forty times greater than if you weren't.

Interestingly, early sun exposure has proven to be key, and where you grow up determines the likelihood that you will develop MS. Fifteen years old seems to be the cutoff age. In other words, if you grow up in the tropics and move to a country in the northern latitudes after age fifteen, your risk of developing MS stays low, and conversely, if you grow up in the northern latitudes and move to the tropics after age fifteen, you continue to have a higher risk of developing MS for the rest of your life. While the exact causes of MS remain unknown, researchers believe a lack of vitamin D in early life may prevent the thymus from killing cells that eventually attack the nerves and eliminate the protective, insulating myelin sheath that is wrapped around the nerves that control motor function.

Studies have shown that women who have high levels of 25-vitamin D reduce their risk of developing MS by about 42 percent.

Scandinavians and Celtic people of northern Europe appear to be predisposed to MS, especially those who don't eat a vitamin D-rich diet. As a result of generations of sun deprivation, these populations may have a higher risk of MS. Based on epidemiological studies, scientists hypothesize that a lack of vitamin D from sunlight caused the immune systems of some people living in these northern latitudes to go awry and attack their nervous systems. Confirmation of this theory is found in studies showing that Norwegians who live near the coast and eat a diet high in vitamin D–rich foods have a much lower risk of MS than those who live inland. Because they live at high latitudes, both groups are at risk of not getting enough natural sunlight. On the other hand, there is almost no incidence of MS among Eskimos who live at very high latitudes. This is thought to be because of their traditional vitamin D–rich diet of polar bear liver, seal blubber, and oily fish.

When immune cells, which, again, have vitamin D receptors, are exposed to appropriate amounts of activated vitamin D, some of which is made by the immune cells themselves, they respond by doing the job they should do and not launching attacks against the body they are supposed to protect. Recently, researchers at the University of Oxford and the University of British Columbia have linked vitamin D with a genetic variant that influences the development of multiple sclerosis.

A group led by Dr. Hector DeLuca used lab studies to demonstrate that pretreating mice with activated vitamin D and then trying to trigger the autoimmune response that causes MS resulted in no MS symptoms. This was due to the protective effect of the activated vitamin D. Unfortunately, despite the tantalizing possibility that vitamin D may be the key to treating MS, so far doctors haven't been able to develop an activated vitamin D therapy that effectively slows or halts the progression of the disease in humans (although I have used vitamin D successfully to treat some of the muscle weakness and bone pain caused by vitamin D deficiency in people with MS). Part of the problem is that by the time a person is diagnosed with MS, it's too late to reverse the autoimmune process that causes the nerve damage. Researchers are testing different ways of administering large doses of activated vitamin D to people with MS, but the results have been disappointing. I have found, in a few of my friends and patients with the first symptoms of MS, that they have not had any further episodes of the disease since they began taking 50,000 IU of vitamin D_2 or its equivalent every two weeks, which is positive.

We're still holding out hope that one day we will develop a method of treating MS with activated vitamin D that can help the millions of people worldwide who have this devastating disease. Until then, it is reasonable to suggest that you can lessen your own and your children's risk of developing MS by getting enough sun exposure to build appropriate levels of 25-vitamin D and, failing that, taking a supplement with enough vitamin D in it to meet your minimum daily needs (refer to part II for guidelines). This is especially important if you grew up in the northern latitudes or are of Scandinavian or Celtic heritage.

Type 1 diabetes (also called juvenile diabetes or insulin-dependent diabetes mellitus) is a chronic disease that occurs when the special pancreatic cells called beta islet cells, which are responsible for making the hormone insulin, are attacked and eventually destroyed by the immune system. This condition is different from type 2, or "adult onset," diabetes, which occurs in adulthood and is not a disease of the immune system. In type 1 diabetes, the pancreas can't produce enough insulin to regulate blood sugar levels and eventually can't produce any insulin at all because all the beta islet cells have been destroyed. This disease almost always occurs in childhood. Although it is acknowledged to be an autoimmune disease, the causes of type 1 diabetes are still considered to be unknown.

Without enough insulin, glucose builds up in the bloodstream instead of entering the cells. The body can't use the glucose for energy, despite high levels in the bloodstream. This causes symptoms such as excessive thirst, frequent need to urinate, and hunger. Five to ten years after the onset of diabetes, the beta islet cells are destroyed and the pancreas is unable to make any insulin at all. Severe conditions, including blindness, kidney failure, hypertension, and heart disease, are among the

regrettable complications of type 1 diabetes. Circulation may deterio-
rate to the extent that ulcers on the legs don't heal, and amputations of
the foot or legs may be necessary.

About fifteen thousand new cases of type 1 diabetes mellitus are diagnosed
each year in the United States, making it the second-most-common chronic
disease in children after asthma. It has been estimated that 1.5 million
people have type 1 diabetes in the United States.

Although epidemiological studies have long suggested that vitamin
D from sun exposure provides immunity to diabetes, a study done in
Finland rocked the medical establishment and confirmed what many
of us believed about the relationship between vitamin D and this disease. Northern Finns experience only two hours of sunlight on Decem-
ber days, and Finland has the world's highest reported incidence of
type 1 diabetes. The study followed more than twelve thousand babies
born in 1966. Those who were given a vitamin D supplement of 2,000
IU a day during the first year of life had a nearly 80 percent reduced
risk of developing diabetes compared with babies who did not receive
a supplement. The study's lead researcher, Dr. Elina Hyppönen, followed the medical records of these children for thirty-one years. Those
who were vitamin D deficient and had rickets had a 2.4-fold risk of
developing type 1 diabetes. In 2008, the Garland brothers were part
of a team of researchers who analyzed the pattern of diabetes in the
world according to latitude and strength of solar UVB radiation. Their
results further confirmed this geographical trend in diabetes. People
who live in sunny climates tend to have a lower risk of type 1 diabetes. Conversely, regions with limited amounts of sunlight have a higher
incidence of diabetes. This disease is very rare in equatorial regions.
They also confirmed that children whose mothers had poor vitamin D
status or who themselves lacked vitamin D had a higher risk of type 1
diabetes.

We know that activated vitamin D may help prevent type 1 diabetes by making the beta islet cells more resistant to attack from the

immune system and by enhancing insulin output by these cells. It can also improve the health of the immune system as a whole, making it less likely that it will malfunction and attack the beta islet cells in the first place. What we don't know, though, is whether a future cure for type 1 diabetes will entail activated vitamin D or this vitamin in a cocktail with other substances. As with MS, the challenge is reversing the course of the immune system once it has already gone off course. In other words, preventing disease from happening in the first place is ideal, and adequate vitamin D may help in the prevention of certain conditions.

Taming the Flames of Rheumatoid Arthritis

Scientists began testing the effects of vitamin D on rheumatoid arthritis (RA) in the 1940s, but initial overdoses caused testing to be suspended until renewed interest arose in the 1990s. Why was there renewed interest? Because we now better understood the role of activated vitamin D on cellular health and had much more efficient and safer ways of administering vitamin D treatment, it became reasonable to revisit the prospect of using vitamin D to treat RA.

Rheumatoid arthritis is a chronic inflammatory disease that primarily affects the joints but can also affect other organ systems. Although the disease can strike a person at any age, it usually comes on between the ages of twenty-five and fifty-five. The disease is more common in older people. Women are affected almost three times as often as men. Between 1 percent and 2 percent of Americans have RA. The rate of advance and severity of the illness varies a great deal from person to person.

The areas of the body most commonly affected by rheumatoid arthritis are the wrists, knees, elbows, fingers, toes, ankles, and neck. Individuals with RA experience bilateral joint pain, joint stiffness, joint warmth, and joint swelling. Other common symptoms include the following:

- fatigue
- discomfort

- appetite loss
- mild fever
- morning stiffness for more than one hour
- joint deformities in the hands and feet
- round, painless nodules under the skin
- skin redness or inflammation
- eye irritation and discharge
- numbness and/or tingling

When a person gets RA, the immune system attacks the lining of the joints, a substance known as synovium, which then becomes inflamed. The process is usually bilateral, which means it affects both knees, both wrists, and so on. Symptoms include pain, swelling, and stiffness of the joints that can lead to joint deformity. These symptoms distinguish rheumatoid arthritis from osteoarthritis, which is a more common and degenerative "wear-and-tear" arthritis.

Complications of RA can be very severe and may include joint destruction, heart failure, lung disease, anemia, low or high platelets, eye disease, cervical (neck) spine instability, neuropathy, and vasculitis (inflammation of blood vessels).

There are no known ways to prevent RA, although the disease's progression can be slowed with early detection and aggressive treatment. Current treatment focuses on reducing inflammation of the joints with anti-inflammatory or immunosuppressive medications such as prednisone, methotrexate, and Enbrel. Unfortunately, most of the successful pharmacological treatments have serious side effects, from life-threatening gastrointestinal bleeding to osteoporosis. Infections also may occur because of the suppression of the immune system. Millions upon millions of dollars are being spent to develop effective treatments for RA that do not have serious side effects.

Studies are currently under way examining how vitamin D may alleviate RA. Preliminary studies suggest that activated vitamin D may be an effective treatment for RA. Mice with RA that were given activated vitamin D experienced a diminishment of the cellular activity responsible for this immune disease, giving rise to the expectation that there may come a day when we can successfully treat RA with injections of activated vitamin D or oral activated vitamin D pills.

Putting Psoriasis in Its Proper Place

Back to psoriasis, the semiautoimmune disease that may be getting wrongly billed as a full-fledged autoimmune disease. Here's my thinking.

Plaque psoriasis is a chronic skin disease that humankind has known about for millennia (the word *psoriasis* is the ancient Greek word for *itch*). Today this disease affects 5.5 million people in the United States and 50 million people worldwide. The condition mostly affects adults, and the symptoms can be extremely distressing, both physically and psychologically.

The characteristic symptoms of psoriasis are raised patches of thick, red skin covered with silvery scales. These unsightly patches, sometimes called plaques, generally itch and may burn. Psoriasis usually occurs on the elbows, knees, scalp, lower back, face, palms, and soles of the feet, but it can affect skin anywhere on the body. In areas such as the knees and elbows, the skin may crack. The disease sometimes affects the fingernails, the toenails, and the flesh inside the mouth. About 15 percent of people with psoriasis have joint inflammation, which produces a crippling form of arthritis called psoriatic arthritis.

Under normal circumstances, skin cells grow, divide, and replace themselves in an orderly fashion, but with psoriasis, cells start reproducing out of control. Psoriatic skin may "turn over" (be replaced) in as little as four days, compared with normal skin, which turns over in twenty-eight days. This rapid turnover, combined with altered maturation of skin cells, results in the characteristic symptoms of psoriasis.

Long before doctors established that psoriasis would respond to directed vitamin D therapy, people with psoriasis knew that their condition improved in response to sun exposure. Folk remedies for psoriasis invariably included sunbaths. One of the first modern medical breakthroughs in treating psoriasis with UV radiation was made in the 1920s by the German doctor William Goeckerman. Goeckerman theorized that, because sunlight helped lessen the symptoms of psoriasis, increasing the intensity of the sun's radiation on the skin of a person who had psoriasis could increase the healthy effects of the sun. He applied a solution of coal tar to the affected areas of skin and then subjected those areas to the radiation of a sunlamp. The coal tar did indeed intensify the effect of the sun's radiation and reduced the symptoms of psoriasis even more than did UV radiation alone. Versions of Goeckerman's treatment of psoriasis are still used today by many dermatologists, who believe that coal tar is still the most effective sensitizing agent for the sun's radiation. UVB irradiation also has been effectively used to treat psoriasis.

More common for severe psoriasis, though, are oral medications that make a patient's skin highly sensitive to sunlight and carefully controlled exposure to UVA radiation at a dermatology clinic (a treatment called psoralen UVA photochemotherapy, or PUVA). Over the years, more than thirty skin diseases have been shown to respond positively to PUVA treatment. This treatment is very effective, but PUVA therapy is quite inconvenient for the patient, who has to visit the clinic two or three times a week. Also, when done too many times, PUVA causes nonmelanoma skin cancer, melanomas, and cataracts. For that reason PUVA is now considered outdated by some.

Until recently, treatment for psoriasis was based on the premise that the disease of psoriasis starts with a defective immune system. I don't believe this to be the case and stated my claim in an editorial in the journal *Experimental Dermatology*. My research shows that although the immune system is certainly involved, the problem begins with a defect in the skin cells themselves. This defect causes the skin cells to reproduce out of control. Only after the skin cells start overproducing does the autoimmune system sense there's something wrong and get involved, which only causes the problem to get worse.

In other words, in psoriasis the autoimmune response is *secondary* to the initial problem in the skin cells. Most treatments for psoriasis were designed to suppress the autoimmune system. Not only does this not address the root cause of the problem—a defect in the skin cells that causes them to reproduce out of control—but it can also have serious side effects. Medications to suppress the autoimmune system, such as cyclosporine, prednisone, and methotrexate, can raise blood pressure, damage the kidneys and liver, and cause osteoporosis, and topical steroids thin the skin (sometimes permanently). Suppressing the body's autoimmune system may also open the door to infection and skin cancer.

A first-line therapy for treating psoriasis is a treatment I helped develop. As detailed at the beginning of this chapter, I discovered that by applying to the affected skin an ointment containing activated vitamin D it was possible to dramatically reduce the symptoms of psoriasis. Galderma Laboratories' Vectical (whose generic name is calcitriol) ointment is the form of activated vitamin D currently available on the market. Another topical drug that developed as a natural progression of my research is Dovonex (calcipotriene), which is an analog of activated vitamin D. This approach of using activated vitamin D and its analogs differs from previous treatments: instead of suppressing the autoimmune response to skin-cell defects, it corrects the skin-cell defects themselves.

Unlike other forms of treatment for psoriasis, activated vitamin D and calcipotriene have no serious side effects (mild skin irritation may occur in sensitive areas). Patients apply the ointment or cream twice a day for six to eight weeks, and the vast majority experience moderate to good results within a matter of weeks. Sometimes these treatments are used in conjunction with a variety of other oral and topical medications, as well as exposure to UVB radiation from the sun or a sunlamp. Another more recent option is Vectical, from the drug company Galderma, which specifically serves the dermatology community. Vectical delivers three micrograms of calcitriol (activated vitamin D) per one gram of ointment and is available by prescription.

Can sunlight alone be used to treat psoriasis? Sunlight is, after all, a main source of vitamin D, and people with psoriasis seem to fare better during the summer months, when it's sunnier. If I see someone who has a mild case of psoriasis and never gets any natural sunlight, I advise the individual to spend more time in the sun to find out whether this alone is enough to treat the symptoms. If this measure is successful, then I advise the person to use an indoor-tanning facility during the nonsunny months (under specific guidelines, though, that you'll read about in chapter 8). If the condition does not improve, the individual should seek the services of a dermatologist experienced in treating psoriasis.

Along with other researchers, my colleagues and I found that the skin has the enzymatic machinery to activate vitamin D, the substance that most effectively prevents unhealthy cell reproduction of the sort characteristic of psoriasis. This may be the explanation for why sun exposure and UVB irradiation are so effective in treating psoriasis.

Everything but the Kitchen Sink

The fact that your immune cells possess vitamin D receptors explains why vitamin D has been shown to influence a spectrum of illnesses blamed on specific infections. Take, for example, tuberculosis. At the turn of the last century, solaria were set up specifically for TB patients. We have always known that macrophages—germ-killing cells of the immune system—activate vitamin D. But we never understood why they did so until recently, when Dr. Robert Modlin's and Dr. John Adams's teams at UCLA revealed that the reason macrophages activate vitamin D is that activated vitamin D tells the macrophage to make cathelicidin, a protein that specifically kills infective agents such as TB.

Their work was published in *Science* in 2006, shedding light on what we had known for more than a century: sunlight can treat tuberculosis. So we now are beginning to realize why vitamin D is so important to innate immunity, especially against infectious agents we can contract in our environment. A study of postmenopausal women who took 2,000 IU of vitamin D a day showed that they had a 90 percent reduction in upper-respiratory-tract infections compared to women who took just 400 IU of vitamin D a day. This study is supported by other observations that risk of upper-respiratory-tract infection is reduced in adults who have the highest circulating blood levels of 25-vitamin D. Extending this observation to other related infections, we can surmise that vitamin D may have an impact on whether you become infected with influenza, which, as I write this, is circling the globe in a new strain called H1N1, or swine flu. Is it possible that just correcting vitamin D deficiency could decrease your risk of contracting the flu to begin with? I think it behooves all of us to be aware of our vitamin D status.

During the 1916 flu epidemic, if you were exposed to influenza, you were less likely to die if you lived in Texas than if you lived in the Northeast.

In 2009, Dr. William Grant presented a hypothesis in an article for *Dermato-Endocrinology* stating that low levels of vitamin D are a risk factor for sepsis, a serious blood condition usually brought on by invading bacteria. That same year, a group at the University of Pittsburgh published a study stating that vitamin D deficiency is associated with bacterial vaginosis, a highly prevalent vaginal infection that plagues many women and can lead to complications during pregnancy.

You might recall a seemingly weird connection made a few years ago between gum disease and heart attacks. On the surface, it's an odd pairing: how can an oral infection or inflammation (periodontitis) cause a heart attack? When you connect the dots from the mouth to the cardiovascular system, you can see how this can happen. One theory is that bacteria in the mouth can affect the heart when they enter the bloodstream. From there, the bacteria can attach to fatty plaques in the heart's blood vessels and contribute to the formation of a clot. Once those blood clots get big enough to obstruct the flow of blood, nutrients and oxygen get restricted and the heart begins to decline in performance. Eventually, a heart attack can occur. Another theory is that the inflammation that accompanies the periodontal disease increases the plaque buildup, which then causes arteries to swell. People with periodontal disease are almost twice as likely to suffer from coronary artery disease as those without periodontal disease.

So how does vitamin D fit in here? Because vitamin D has the power to assist the body's natural defense against bad bacteria and inflammation, keeping healthy levels of 25-vitamin D (so that the immune cells can activate it) ultimately reduces the risk of this chain of events happening. The mechanism is the same as the one for tuberculosis: 1,25-vitamin D promotes the production of a protein (cathelicidin) that fights bacterial infections in the mouth.

Tooth decay (cavities) and periodontal disease are linked to low 25-vitamin D levels.

This also explains why dental cavities (tooth decay) have been associated with vitamin D deficiency. As most people know, dental cavities are more common among younger people (below the age of fifty) and periodontal disease is more common in older people. We were aware of a connection between sunlight exposure and the prevalence of cavities as far back as the 1930s, when an ecological study reported an inverse relationship between mean hours of sunlight and the presence of tooth decay in boys aged twelve to fourteen years living in rural or semirural regions of the United States. In other words, more sunlight exposure correlated with fewer cavities. There was a general increase in cavities, going from 2.9 cavities per boy for those living where there were more than 3,000 hours of sunshine a year to 4.9 cavities per boy for those living where there were less than 2,200 hours of sunshine a year.

The anti-inflammatory quality of vitamin D explains why it's been associated with the prevention and treatment of asthma and allergic reactions. It has also been touted as a great addition to steroid-based treatments for asthmatics who typically don't respond well to traditional steroid inhalers or tablets. When vitamin D is added to a steroid regimen in these patients, the immune system responds as T cells synthesize a molecule called IL-10. This molecule, which acts as a signal, can inhibit the immune responses that cause the symptoms of allergic and asthmatic disease. Later on, when I cover a few pregnancy issues, you'll see that vitamin D's immunological power can play a significant role in preventing a lifetime of allergic diseases in unborn children. The power of vitamin D to support the immune system is proof again that it serves a profound function in our lives from start to finish.

I believe we're just beginning to understand the power of vitamin D in preserving and enhancing the immune system. Just before this book went to press, more studies emerged showing that vitamin D can boost the production of proactive compounds in the skin itself and may ultimately help prevent skin infections, particularly those caused by microbial invasions. But that's just scratching the surface, so to speak. Vitamin D, as you know by now, responds to receptors all over the body and in its deepest cells and tissues. To say vitamin D has anti-inflammatory, antimicrobial, antiviral, anti-*anything* properties is an understatement. Vitamin D may be one of our most reliable *pro*active ingredients in bolstering comprehensive immunity and reinforcing the body's natural defenses.

In the next chapter, we'll make a departure from the immune system but see that vitamin D serves an equally comprehensive role in aiding matters of the mind, including emotions.

CHAPTER 6

Mind Matters and Mixed Emotions

The facts of light on mood, mental states,
and sense of well-being

A voiding the sun can sometimes feel like you're trying to avoid eating a freshly baked chocolate-chip cookie when you're watching your diet. Something in your brain starts talking to you, triggering you to (quite subconsciously) take a small bite of the cookie, or, in this case, let your body be exposed to a little sunshine (just a few seconds won't hurt!). It tastes—and feels—delicious. You can't stop eating the cookie. You can't stop soaking up some rays. Bites become the whole thing. Seconds turn into minutes. Is there a reason why the sun can feel so good?

That sense of well-being after exposure to UV radiation is very physical and probably has been ingrained in our DNA for longer than we've been human. Sun exposure provides a natural high by stimulating the release of "feel-good" substances in your body, such as serotonin, dopamine, and beta endorphins, the body's natural opiate. (An equivalent response can be obtained from eating the cookie, as some of those same hormones get released—contributing to that all-too-familiar rush of euphoria.) Sunshine also suppresses hormones like melatonin, which make you feel sluggish and "down." We used to think that this release of hormones had to begin in the hypothalamus, our brain's command center for emotions and the origin of countless hormonal reactions. But recently scientists have unlocked the secret messaging service that takes place right there in your skin cells. It turns out our skin and nervous system share a language we are just beginning to understand. We now know, for example, that those hormones key to mood may not originate only in the brain. They can be created by skin cells upon exposure to UV radiation and then enter the bloodstream and travel to the brain. Now that's a two-way street.

Sunshine has more than a short-term impact on your psychological state. It almost completely controls the biological tempo of your life— your daily pattern of body temperature highs and lows, levels of alertness, sleeping patterns, hormonal secretions, and other basic biological functions, such as when you eat. It may even factor into your risk of dementia later in life. Let's take a look at these connections. Along the way I'll call out further connections that involve vitamin D.

Your Biological Clock

Biological clocks, while sometimes pigeonholed as referring mainly to a woman's reproductive time frame, tick in all humans and don't have anything to do with procreation. Everyone has what's called a circadian rhythm, characterized by a cycle of changes your body undergoes every day. Much of this rhythm is carefully controlled by the ebb and flow of hormones throughout your day, which factor into things like your sleep, appetite, and energy levels. Until the early 1980s, scientists believed humans had evolved to a point where we controlled our own circadian rhythms. But we've uncovered a lot more about our bodies since then, and only in the past few years have scientists begun to understand how our circadian rhythm affects our ability to think and act. And it's not a rhythm that beats to the drum of our willful wants and desires.

While it could be nice to have a biological clock fully under our own conscious control and subject to our personal commands, circadian rhythms answer to sunshine. Our biological clock is kept on a twenty-four-hour schedule by the rise and fall of light. Without sunshine and darkness signals, your sleep/wake schedule would shift forward by an hour every day—or "free run"—as it does in submariners, astronauts, and anyone else who lives without regular exposure to natural sunlight. How does this mechanism work? It's really quite intriguing.

Your biological clock is made up of a small cluster of cells called the suprachiasmatic nucleus (SCN), which is located near the center of the brain. Sunlight hits the photoreceptors in the retina of your eye, and this signal travels via the optic nerve to the hypothalamus, your brain's emotional headquarters, where the SCN is located. In addition to housing the SCN, the hypothalamus is responsible for a variety of involuntary functions that control your mood.

One of the most important jobs of the hypothalamus is to send signals to the pineal gland, a pea-sized structure known as the third eye located deep between the hemispheres of your brain (it looks like a tiny pinecone—hence its name). When it is dark outside, the gland releases a substance called melatonin, which makes your system slow down and prepares you for sleep. Conversely, when the SCN receives signals that light is around, it sends messages to the pineal gland to shut down production of melatonin and increase production of serotonin, which makes you feel happy and alert.

How can we be so biologically influenced by the sun? When our ancestors were first evolving, humans lived by the rise and fall of the sun. In other words, without electricity and a way to work past nightfall, people slowed down after sunset and rested for the next day. Thus, our physiology evolved in such a way as to shut down when darkness began and start up in response to sunlight. It isn't just the sleep-wake cycle that is affected by your circadian rhythms; a variety of other psychological and physical functions are profoundly influenced as well. Many people who suffer from sleep problems have an internal clock that has become out of sync or mismatched with the day-night cycle. That is to say, their bodies' physiologies don't mesh with society's twenty-four-hour clock.

Everyone's circadian clock or "pacemaker" ticks at a different rate. And, in fact, a team of German scientists in 2008 discovered that you can look at your skin cell genes to determine whether you are a lark (who likes to get up early) or an owl (who likes to stay up late). Our preferences for rising early or late are encoded in our genes, including those found in skin cells. These scientists engineered a way to observe and measure individual "clocks" in human skin cells. After taking skin samples from volunteers, they inserted into each cell a gene that lights up in ultraviolet light when the cell is metabolically most active. The gene allowed the scientists to follow the circadian rhythm of the cells as they changed over a twenty-four-hour period. In essence, they were able to identify and track skin cells' built-in timing mechanism set by the central biological clock of the body. This is possible because most cell types have a genetic imprint of a person's unique circadian physiology.

You may not give much thought to your circadian rhythm. You probably take for granted that you will be sleepy at night and then feel awake and alert during the day. Your mood may vary, but you manage to navigate life's semipaved road. Some days you may wake up on the wrong side of the bed, but for the most part you are reasonably good-humored.

Science is still trying to understand completely how our body clocks work, and even how many body clocks we have. In addition to the clock set by cues of day and night, we also have a neurological clock that has an internal schedule set in the brain. When these two clocks don't agree on the same schedule and compete with one another, we feel "off," which is what happens with classic jet lag. If your circadian rhythm is synchronized with your daily life, then chances are your mood state will be a vibrant one. However, millions of people have circadian rhythm dysfunction, and they experience mood-related problems such as seasonal affective disorder and other forms of depression, premenstrual syndrome, and sleeping disorders characterized by not being able to sleep enough, sleeping too much, or not being able to sleep at the right time. If you have what's called delayed sleep phase syndrome, for example, your clock is set *later*. You may find it difficult to fall asleep until the early hours of the morning—sometimes two or three o'clock—and may not be alert until noontime or later. People with advanced sleep phase syndrome have a biological clock that is set *earlier* than their natural environment. They tend to feel groggy and tired in the afternoon, fall asleep in the very early evening, then wake up in the middle of the night without being able to fall back to sleep.

Sometimes the cure for simple circadian rhythm imbalances is to hit your "reset" button by exposure to light (preferably bright morning light) and by activity. This will help synchronize your biological clock that beats to the tune of daylight versus nighttime and your neurological clock. For example, when you want to be alert and awake but your body doesn't want to follow, you can stimulate your body to reset itself just by going outside into the sunlight for ten or fifteen minutes or engaging in some physical activity, preferably outside in the bright light.

Circadian rhythm disorders are also thought to be associated with physical illnesses, including heart disease and gastrointestinal disorders. Based on our growing understanding of the importance of sunshine on the functioning of the biological clock, scientists are now able to successfully treat most circadian rhythm–related conditions using artificial bright light.

Mood Therapy Through Sunlight

Spending more time in the sun to improve your circadian rhythm health may also improve your vitamin D status, but the bright-light treatments that are at the heart of modern treatment of circadian rhythm disorders will not increase the vitamin D in your bloodstream. Not only is your biological clock set by light hitting your *eyes*—not your skin—but the kind of light your body prefers for calibrating its clock is early-morning light. At this time of day, too little UVB radiation is penetrating the atmosphere to also get a good dose of vitamin D.

In addition to scheduling morning exposure to sunlight to help keep the biological clock ticking in time with the twenty-four-hour day, one of the most common methods used today to address circadian rhythm disorders is the light box. Light boxes emit up to 10,000 lux (a measurement of light intensity) and mimic natural sunshine at around noontime. The light emitted by these devices is twenty times the intensity of average indoor light (500 to 1,000 lux), which, most people are surprised to find out, is only as strong as the natural twilight.

The light boxes themselves consist of a set of fluorescent bulbs installed in a box with a diffusing screen that spreads the light evenly and filters out all UVB and most UVA radiation. Using a light box is easy. You simply position the box on a nearby table or desktop and sit comfortably for the treatment session. It's imperative to sit or stand close to the light box, with or without the room lights on, and your eyes must be open. Looking directly at the lights is unnecessary; instead, light-box users pass the time reading, writing, watching TV, or eating a meal. The only reported side effects are occasional slight headaches. The duration of bright-light treatment sessions varies from fifteen minutes to three hours a day, depending on your individual needs and the equipment you use. The more powerful the unit, the less time you have to spend in front of it to get the same effect. Also, the nearer you are to the light source, the higher the intensity of light shining through your eyes and the quicker and more effective the treatment.

The timing of light treatments is extremely important and varies with each person, depending on the type of circadian rhythm disorder being addressed. People who have late-night insomnia, for example, and thus have trouble getting up in the morning after going to bed too late, may only need one brief treatment a day in the morning to speed the body clock up; those with early-morning insomnia have the reverse problem—they wake up too early and fall asleep in the early evening. These people need to slow down their body clocks and can typically do so with early evening sessions of bright-light therapy to avert their superearly bedtimes and align their bodies with the twenty-four-hour day. Knowing exactly what kind of rhythm disorder you may have and then scheduling the right kind of light therapy is important, and this reinforces the need to use bright-light treatment under the supervision of a qualified sleep therapist.

You don't need a prescription for a light box, but anyone suffering from a serious mood-related disorder should certainly seek a doctor's recommendation before obtaining a unit and use it under the doctor's supervision. Choose your doctor wisely, and question one who only prescribes drugs such as sedatives or antidepressants for your condition. Some doctors are unaware of the successful results of bright light therapy.

Several reputable companies sell light boxes (see the Resource Guide on page 269). The key to successful bright-light treatment is using a product that provides strong light at a reasonable unit-to-user distance. It is important that you purchase your light box from a trusted company, because there's no way you can measure the lux output of a bright-light unit. If your symptoms don't improve, you won't know if it is because the inexpensive light box you bought is not emitting strong enough light or because your condition is resistant to bright-light treatment. Tests of products sold by disreputable companies demonstrate that certain light boxes don't put out the amount of light they are advertised as emitting. Also, poor-quality screens may not filter out enough UV radiation, which may damage your eyes. A portable unit might suit you if you travel a lot, or one with a stand may fit your needs if you plan to get bright-light treatment while working out on a treadmill or stair climber. Numerous accessories are also available, including padded carrying cases and stands that let you place the light box in different positions. These units can cost between two hundred and seven hundred dollars, depending on a variety of factors, the most important being the unit's lux output and the distance it can project that light intensity. Many insurance companies will reimburse the purchase price of light fixtures for the treatment of seasonal affective disorder, PMS, and sleep disorders.

Seasonal Affective Disorder (SAD)

If you live at a higher latitude, you are probably aware of some minor changes in yourself that accompany the lengthening days of late fall and winter. Because there's less light—in terms of both intensity and duration—your hibernation impulse makes you want to eat more and be less energetic. Most of us cope quite well with these changes, and indeed, some become energized by the prospect of brisk January days and winter sports.

However, a significant number of people are extremely sensitive to changes in the length of the day, so much so that for them living a normal life in the modern age is difficult. In winter, their biological clocks tell them to hibernate, even though life tells them they have work to do, meetings to attend, prime-time television shows to watch, and kids to feed. Most of these people find it difficult to fulfill the everyday demands of life during the winter months.

This syndrome has been known for millennia. Hippocrates identified it in the time of the ancient Greeks. On May 16, 1898, Arctic voyager Dr. Frederick Cook wrote poignantly of psychological changes his fellow explorers were experiencing in response to the lack of sunlight:

> The winter and the darkness have slowly but steadily settled over us. . . . It is not difficult to read on the faces of my companions their thoughts and moody dispositions. . . . The curtain of blackness which has fallen over the outer world of icy desolation has also descended upon the inner world of our souls. Around the tables . . . men are sitting about sad and dejected, lost in dreams of melancholy from which, now and then, one arouses with an empty attempt at enthusiasm. For brief moments some try to break the spell by jokes, told perhaps for the fiftieth time. Others grind out a cheerful philosophy, but all efforts to infuse bright hopes fail.

This condition was formally identified in 1984 by Dr. Norman Rosenthal of the National Institute of Mental Health and was given the name seasonal affective disorder, or SAD (a highly appropriate acronym). Rosenthal established that this was a bona fide disorder by taking a group of people who reported serious symptoms of "winter depression" and tracking them through the various seasons. With startling accuracy, he showed that their symptoms worsened with the shortening days and improved as the days got longer. Since Rosenthal's landmark study, many other researchers have confirmed his findings.

How Do You Know If You Have SAD?

The characteristic symptom of SAD is the onset of major depressive feelings at certain times of the year. Physical activity decreases. You feel very lethargic and even sluggish. Almost any physical activity seems to be too much effort. On the other hand, your appetite increases and you have a particular craving for carbohydrates and sugars, such as starches, pastries, and other sweets, and alcohol. This explains why people with SAD usually put on weight during the winter. Most people with SAD sleep for long hours—or wish they could! They may lose interest in sex, become irritable and bad tempered, and have trouble thinking clearly and quickly, which may lead to mistakes.

Symptoms of SAD

The "blahs" or "cabin fever" are not the same as SAD. Symptoms of full-blown SAD include the following:

- depression that begins in fall or winter

- lack of energy

- decreased interest in work or important activities

- increased appetite with weight gain

- carbohydrate and sugar cravings

- increased need for sleep and excessive daytime sleepiness

- social withdrawal

- extreme afternoon slumps with decreased energy and concentration

- decreased sex drive

Epidemiologists estimate that 2 percent to 3 percent of Americans develop full-blown SAD, with another 7 percent suffering a less extreme form of this condition. Women are four times as likely to get SAD, and the average age of onset is twenty-three. Because winter days are shorter at higher latitudes, the farther you live from the equator the greater the chance you'll develop SAD. About 1.5 percent of people who live in Florida get SAD, while this condition afflicts almost 10 percent of people in New Hampshire.

The term *holiday blues* has been used to describe SAD. That's because in the Northern Hemisphere, the onset of SAD symptoms begins when people are gearing up for Thanksgiving, Christmas, and the New Year, and the omnipresent good cheer contrasts with many people's "blue mood." Until Dr. Rosenthal published his study, many people thought the holiday season itself was responsible for arousing depressive feelings in those who couldn't be with their loved ones or who felt stress in anticipation of family get-togethers.

What exactly is happening to people who develop SAD? I described earlier how darkness causes the pineal gland to release melatonin to make us slow down and go to sleep. Winter wreaks havoc with some people's physiology, and unlike the rest of us, individuals with SAD aren't able to suppress the production of melatonin in their system caused by the dim winter light.

SAD is a major depressive syndrome with clinical manifestations. Thanks to the pioneering work of doctors like Norman Rosenthal, it is now listed in the American Psychiatric Association's standard text, the Diagnostic and Statistical Manual of Mental Disorders. In the past, SAD has been treated using strong antidepressant drugs and even electric shock therapy. However, by far the most effective treatment for SAD is sunlight, or artificial bright light that replicates the effect of sunshine in the summer. In Norman Rosenthal's study, he told a large group of patients that he was going to expose them to bright light, which might or might not help their condition. He exposed half the patients to the kind of high-intensity light that simulates midday summer sunshine (between 5,000 and 10,000 lux) and the rest to the equivalent to bright indoor household light (bright office lighting emits between 500 and 700 lux, which is equal only to the light at dusk or dawn). The patients did not know which type of light therapy they were getting. Almost all the SAD patients who were exposed to the high-intensity lights experienced a dramatic reduction in symptoms, whereas those in the yellow-light group saw no improvement. Numerous studies have duplicated these results. Bright-light treatment administered by a light box is now the treatment of choice if you have SAD. 80 percent of people with SAD benefit from it. Remember, it's important to have a qualified doctor provide you with guidelines for using your light box, although you will find through trial and error what works best for you.

Therapists usually have their SAD patients start with a single ten- to fifteen-minute session every day, gradually increasing their exposure to thirty to forty-five minutes. If symptoms persist or worsen as the days shorten, two sessions a day may be the protocol—one in the morning, upon waking, and another in the evening. As with any bright-light treatment, however, figuring out the ideal timing to treat a specific condition should be done under the care of a doctor or therapist trained in this arena. Total daily exposure is usually limited to between ninety minutes and two hours. Keep in mind that the light boxes used to treat SAD are not sunlamps, so you will not get a tan from them—nor any vitamin D benefits. Studies have shown that morning bright-light sessions work better to treat the symptoms of SAD.

The Clinical Practice Guidelines issued by the U.S. Department of Health and Human Services recognize bright light as a generally accepted treatment for SAD. However, on the rare occasion that bright-light treatments don't work, antidepressant medications may be prescribed for use in conjunction with this kind of therapy.

SAD symptoms usually improve after just a few days of bright-light therapy. The best results are seen in people who stick to a consistent schedule beginning in the fall or winter and continuing until the spring. A common mistake is to discontinue treatments as soon as you feel better. In such cases, the symptoms return. This reinforces the need to keep up treatments throughout the winter months.

Guidelines for Minimizing the "Winter Blahs"

If your spirits inevitably sink a little during the winter months, you may have not seasonal affective disorder but a less serious, or subclinical, version of this condition colloquially referred to as the winter blahs. Be attuned to your moods and energy levels. If you start feeling "low" toward the end of summer, take preventive action, including some of the following measures:

• Get as much natural sunlight as possible. When it's sunny, spend as much time as you can outdoors. Early-morning sunlight is ideal, as this can help calibrate a circadian rhythm gone haywire.

• If you are at home during the day, keep the curtains open as much as possible.

• If you work in an office, try to get a workspace that's near a window.

• Be physically active, and begin your physical activity before the symptoms start. Physical activity outside in the bright morning light is a win-win.

• Try to establish a mind-set that will enable you to enjoy the wintertime. Plan active events for yourself in advance of the fall. Schedule things to look forward to.

If you feel yourself succumbing, don't feel ashamed or try to hide it. You are by no means alone. Seek competent professional help. What you learn this winter you can apply in winters to come.

Nonseasonal Depression

There are different degrees of nonseasonal depression.

Mild depression, or the "blues," may be brought on by an unhappy event, such as a divorce or the death of a relative, and is characterized by feelings of sadness, gloominess, or emptiness, which may be accompanied by lethargy.

Chronic low-grade depression, also known as dysthymia, exists when a person feels depressed most of the time for a period of two years. These feelings are accompanied by changes in energy, appetite, or sleep, as well as low self-esteem and feelings of hopelessness.

Major depression involves severe, persistent mood depression and loss of interest and pleasure in daily activities, accompanied by decreased energy, changes in sleep and appetite, and feelings of guilt or hopelessness. These symptoms must be present for at least two weeks, cause significant distress, and be severe enough to interfere with functioning. If the depression is very severe, it may be accompanied by psychotic symptoms or by suicidal thoughts or behaviors.

Until recently, few studies had measured the effect of bright light on nonseasonal depression. The success of bright-light treatment on seasonal affective disorder, however, has prompted numerous researchers to study whether this therapy would be effective for the treatment of nonseasonal depression. The results have been extremely encouraging.

Several studies have shown that bright-light therapy alone is as effective as antidepressant medications in reducing the symptoms of nonseasonal depression. One study showed that just a single hour of bright-light treatment was as effective as several weeks on a standard medication for depression. Some of the most significant work in this area is being done at the University of California at San Diego and at the University of Vienna. Researchers at these institutions have found that combining bright-light therapy and antidepressant medications is an extremely successful way to alleviate the symptoms of depression.

Bright-light therapy is a fundamental component of the latest and most successful treatment for nonseasonal depression. This form of therapy involves a three-pronged approach: bright-light exposure, antidepressant medication, and "wake therapy." In wake therapy, patients wake themselves halfway through the night on the first night their program begins and stay awake until they have their bright-light treatment at around breakfast time (these patients had already begun antidepressant medications, so the effects of the drug had begun). Wake therapy seems to intensify the effectiveness of the bright-light therapy, perhaps because it jump-starts the suppression of melatonin production and increases serotonin production. Patients who have undergone this "triple-whammy" depression therapy have experienced a 27 percent decrease in symptoms in one week.

The success of bright light in treating depressive disorders has inspired doctors to use this therapy to treat conditions such as bulimia, chronic fatigue syndrome, post- and antepartum depression, alcohol withdrawal syndrome, adolescent depression, jet lag, and certain forms of mental illness.

The Vitamin D Link to Depression

While several factors may play into the onset and progression of depression, whether mild or severe, vitamin D deficiency has been shown to contribute to depression and even chronic fatigue. This is due to the fact that activated vitamin D in the adrenal glands helps regulate an enzyme called tyrosine hydroxylase, which is necessary for the production of dopamine, epinephrine, and norepinephrine—those hormones critical to mood, stress management, and energy. The adrenal glands pump these hormones to help us cope with daily stress. Without ample vitamin D to keep the adrenals in check, they can continue to pump these powerful hormones out and the body can begin to experience constant exhaustion that may then lead to chronic fatigue. And there's no doubt that being in a chronic fatigued state can perpetuate feelings of depression.

One insightful study performed in Minneapolis tested for vitamin D deficiency among 150 children and adults at an inner-city primary-care clinic. Many of these people were immigrants from various corners of the globe, and all of them had come into the clinic between February 2000 and June 2002 complaining of vague, nonspecific pain. Among the myriad symptoms recorded by doctors were achy lower-back pain, insomnia, fatigue, weakness, and a depressed mood. Many of them were diagnosed with depression and sent home with nonsteroidal anti-inflammatory drugs (NSAIDs, such as Aleve and Motrin) to help take the edge off their elusive pains, and in some cases, antidepressants were prescribed. I mentioned this study back in chapter 3, but here I want to give you a closer look at the individual profiles of these patients, which turn up some interesting findings with regard to their vitamin D status, their specific ethnicity, and how they were treated.

None of the patients had any known disorder that would prevent them from manufacturing vitamin D in the body, and none had ever been tested for 25-vitamin D. Less than 10 percent were taking a vitamin supplement at the time of the study, and more than 90 percent had been evaluated by a doctor for their persistent musculoskeletal pain one year or more before the screening for 25-vitamin D. A full 93 percent of all these people were shown to have deficient levels of 25-vitamin D. Every single one of the East Africans and Hispanics tested low for 25-vitamin D (specifically, they had 25-vitamin D levels of 20 nanograms per milliliter or less); 89 percent of the Southeast Asians also scored this low. And to the researchers' surprise, all of the African Americans, all of the American Indians, and 83 percent of the white patients were proved to be vitamin D deficient.

Perhaps the most alarming finding of all was what the screening revealed when looked at by age group. The degree of severity of vitamin D deficiency was *inversely* proportionate by age group. The youngest patients showed the lowest 25-vitamin D levels, and of the five who had *undetectable* serum 25-vitamin D levels, four were thirty-five years of age or younger. Many of the patients were given vastly different diagnoses and treatments. A twenty-three-year old white female diagnosed with depression, nondegenerative joint disease, and low-back pain was given over-the-counter and prescription nonsteroidal anti-inflammatories. A fifty-eight-year old African American male, on the other hand, diagnosed with a panoply of health conditions, was given a corresponding panoply of drugs, including narcotics and an antidepressant.

Could any or all of these serious health challenges have been averted had these patients maintained sufficient levels of 25-vitamin D? One thing is certain: people who suffer from persistent, nonspecific pain and who are subsequently diagnosed as showing signs of depression alongside elusive other symptoms like fatigue and insomnia would do well to have their 25-vitamin D levels checked or simply take vitamin D as I prescribe in chapter 10.

Taking Depression Symptoms Seriously

Just because your depression symptoms occur only at certain times of the year doesn't mean they are all in your head. The symptoms of depression—seasonal or nonseasonal—must be taken very seriously.

Proper diagnosis and treatment are essential. If you experience persistent sadness that lasts for more than two weeks, accompanied by problems with sleep, appetite, concentration, and energy, seek professional help. This is especially important if you are experiencing thoughts of suicide or of hurting yourself.

There's no mechanical device to measure depression, so how do doctors tell if antidepression treatments such as bright light are working? Scientists rate how depressed patients are before and after treatment with "depression rating scales." They interview patients and ask them to score how sad, guilty, without appetite, suicidal, and so forth they are, and then they add up the points to reach a total depression score. After therapy, the researchers ask the same questions. If the score is the same or higher, they conclude that the treatment made no difference or perhaps made the patient's condition worse. But if the score is lower, the treatment has worked.

Premenstrual Syndrome (PMS)

Premenstrual syndrome (PMS) refers to a cluster of symptoms that occur regularly in conjunction with a woman's monthly menstrual period. The symptoms tend to occur five to eleven days before her period starts and stop when her period begins.

Most women are affected by PMS at some point during their childbearing years. Between 30 percent and 40 percent of women have PMS symptoms severe enough to interfere with daily living, and 10 percent suffer symptoms so severe they are debilitating. PMS can cause extreme difficulties in a woman's relationships with friends, family, and colleagues.

The incidence of PMS is higher in those between their late twenties and early forties, those with at least one child, those with a family history of a major depression disorder, and those with a past medical history of either postpartum depression or some other affective mood disorder, such as SAD. It used to be thought that PMS symptoms were caused by a hormonal imbalance that occurred during the menstrual cycle. Now it's understood that PMS is a result of insufficient serotonin—the chemical that carries messages between the nerves and makes us feel calm, happy, and alert. Just before a woman gets her period, her levels of serotonin naturally drop and then go back up again when her period starts. If she has naturally low base levels of serotonin, symptoms of PMS will probably occur as serotonin levels drop below the point at which they are needed to maintain good psychological health.

Several researchers have demonstrated that PMS responds well to bright-light treatment. The reason bright light works to reduce the symptoms of PMS is quite straightforward: serotonin levels in the body increase in response to bright light; remember, too, that vitamin D helps regulate the production of dopamine, the other mood-friendly hormone, in the brain. One of the most important studies in the last decade of how bright light can be used to treat PMS was led by Dr. D. J. Anderson and published in the *Journal of Obstetrics and Gynecology*. Dr. Anderson's six-month study involved a group of twenty women who had unsuccessfully tried in a variety of ways to reduce their serious, ongoing problems with PMS. The women were given fifteen to twenty-nine minutes of bright-light therapy every day for four consecutive menstrual periods. At the end of the study, Dr. Anderson and his colleagues found that the bright-light treatments had reduced by 76 percent the severity of PMS symptoms such as depression, anxiety, irritability, poor concentration, fatigue, food cravings, bloating, and breast pain.

There may be a vitamin D link as well. Because ovarian hormones influence calcium, magnesium, and vitamin D metabolism, scientists have long believed that PMS can be partly blamed on low levels of these micronutrients. Dr. Susan Thys-Jacobs of Columbia University published a study in 2000 making a strong case for calcium, highlighting that the addition of not just calcium but also magnesium and vitamin D can completely reverse PMS. A year before that study, Dr. Thys-Jacobs's investigations revealed that polycystic ovarian syndrome also could be corrected by supplementation of vitamin D and calcium. Polycystic ovarian syndrome is a condition in which a woman's hormones become imbalanced, often causing a disruption in her menstrual cycle and infertility. Dr. Thys-Jacobs examined thirteen premenopausal women with a history of abnormal ovulation and related menstrual problems.

Their mean 25-vitamin D levels were 11.2 (yes, that's deficient). After they were treated with calcium therapy and their vitamin D brought up to sufficient levels, seven of the women had normal menstrual cycles within two months, including two who had resolved previously dysfunctional bleeding. Two of the women became pregnant, and the other four patients maintained normal menstrual cycles.

Another side effect of some women's monthly cycle—menstrual migraine—has also been associated with low levels of vitamin D and calcium. Recall that we saw earlier how vitamin D deficiency is common in chronic migraine sufferers; this is aside from the menstrual factor and includes men, too.

Symptoms of Premenstrual Syndrome

You have PMS if five or more of these symptoms are associated with your menstrual period:

- feeling of sadness or hopelessness, possible suicidal thoughts

- feelings of tension or anxiety

- mood swings marked by periods of crying

- persistent irritability or anger that affects other people

- disinterest in daily activities and relationships

- trouble concentrating

- fatigue or low energy

- food cravings or binging

- sleep disturbances

- feelings of being out of control

- Physical symptoms, such as bloating, breast tenderness, headaches, and joint or muscle pain

Shift Worker Syndrome

Tens of millions of Americans work the night shift. Night-shift workers experience a variety of problems, such as a higher risk of psychological ailments and an increased likelihood of fatigue-related accidents. Night workers also have higher rates of heart disease, cancer, diabetes, and gastrointestinal disorders.

Despite the additional expense of paying people to work the night shift and the problems it causes for the workers, in this modern age we need people working unfavorable hours. Certain industries, such as oil refining, shipping, and transportation, need to operate around the clock; others find it economically desirable to keep the assembly line moving; emergency response and law enforcement need personnel operating their stations twenty-four hours a day; and convenience stores need to keep their doors open in case someone needs a gallon of milk at two o'clock in the morning.

Night-shift workers experience problems because their lives operate in opposition to their circadian rhythms. No matter how long a person works the night shift, when he leaves work and walks into the daylight to go home to bed, his body clock tells him it is time to wake up. That makes it hard for that person to get a full night's sleep during the day.

Studies of night-shift workers have shown that, on average, they sleep one to two hours less than day workers. That sleep loss is cumulative and is primarily responsible for the problems night shift workers tend to have staying alert during their shifts and experiencing a fulfilling life outside work. Shift workers also pay a huge toll in their relationships with others and ability to maintain a stable household.

A large number of studies have shown that bright-light therapy is extremely helpful in helping night-shift workers adapt to their work schedules. Companies that have employees working the night shift should fully utilize bright-light technology to improve worker morale and reduce errors and accidents on the job. The keys to this are having the appropriate bright-light equipment installed and timing its use to synchronize workers' body clocks to their working and sleeping hours.

Guidelines for Decreasing Circadian Rhythm Disruptions Caused by Shift Work

• Reduce the number of consecutive night shifts you work. Night-shift workers get less sleep than day workers. Over several days, they become progressively more sleep deprived. If you limit the number of night shifts you work to five or fewer, with days off in between, you are more likely to recover from sleep deprivation. If you work a twelve-hour shift instead of the usual eight hours, limit this to four consecutive shifts. After several consecutive night shifts, you should ideally receive a forty-eight-hour break.

• Avoid working prolonged shifts, working excessive overtime, and taking only short breaks.

• Avoid long commutes, because they waste time you could spend sleeping.

• Avoid rotating shifts more than once a week. It is more difficult to cope with such alteration than it is to work the same shift for extended periods. The sequence of shift rotation can be important as well. Working the first shift, then the second shift, and then the third shift is easier than working the first, the third, and then the second.

• Get enough sleep on your days off. Practice good "sleep hygiene" by planning and arranging a sleep schedule and by avoiding caffeine, alcohol, and nicotine to help you sleep or stay awake.

• Avoid reliance on stimulants, over-the-counter and otherwise. Caffeine and stay-awake pills only temporarily trick the body into thinking it is functioning properly, which will only further disrupt your circadian rhythms.

Sleep Disturbances and Elder Care

Bright light is being used with increasing frequency and success to treat a variety of disorders that affect our older citizens, especially sleep-pattern disturbances and forms of dementia such as Alzheimer's disease.

As people get older, their circadian rhythms "flatten out" and they become predisposed to sleep disturbances. This usually manifests itself in going to sleep too early and then waking before the sun comes up—often at three or four o'clock in the morning. In the most extreme cases, elderly nursing home patients may sleep at any hour of the day or night, sometimes even sleeping for part of every hour in the day. Bright-light therapy first thing in the morning, following the same guidelines used for seasonal affective disorder, has been effective in resetting elderly people's biological clocks and restoring their circadian rhythms. Increasingly, attention is being paid to the kinds of lighting that should be provided for seniors, not just in the form of directed therapy but also as it should be incorporated into the design and architecture of homes and group living facilities.

Sleep Tips

Want a better night's sleep? Try the following:

- Cut down on caffeine (including caffeinated soda) after 2:00 P.M. and avoid alcohol.

- Drink fewer fluids before going to sleep so you won't be awakened by bladder discomfort.

- Avoid heavy meals close to bedtime.

- Avoid nicotine, which acts as a stimulant—not a relaxant.

- Exercise regularly, but do so in the early afternoon, not in the late afternoon or evening.

- Relax in a hot tub or bath before bedtime.

- Establish a regular bedtime and wake-time schedule. Keep to that schedule on the weekends.

If your sleep problems become chronic, consider bright-light therapy. Even people with mild sleeping disorders can benefit from bright-light treatment. For example, a person who wants to go to sleep at eleven in the evening but can't nod off until one in the morning can reset the body's clock by having a leisurely breakfast in front of a light box.

The Future of Treatment for Circadian Rhythm Disorders

Bright-light treatment is an exciting breakthrough in the treatment of mood-related conditions caused by circadian rhythm dysfunction. Treatments are safe and economical, and light boxes have no side effects. Light boxes represent a one-time cost of a few hundred dollars, versus seventy dollars per month for an antidepressant that has side effects and other risks. However, bright-light treatments can be extremely effective when used in conjunction with antidepressant medications in some cases.

Recent breakthroughs have demonstrated that bright "blue light" treatments may have even more applications than we fully understand. Rather than the traditional 10,000-lux full-spectrum light therapy devices, blue-light devices emit exactly what they say: blue light, which is a very specific range of light within the visible spectrum that has a wavelength of 526 nanometers. For some time, blue light treatments have been used with great success for babies with jaundice. More recently, blue light treatments have been used to stimulate weight gain in premature babies. The Department of Architecture at the Massachusetts Institute of Technology is studying how to maximize natural daylight and minimize artificial light in buildings. It is developing tools to measure how illumination can be manipulated to meet human circadian needs in order to help architects make light-related design decisions. A colleague of mine has been at the forefront of creating headlamps that a person can simply put on to be exposed to blue light.

Blue-light therapy can have multiple benefits. One recent study found that using blue light helped office workers stay more alert during the day, reduced evening fatigue, and improved night sleep. Some research suggests this is because blue light targets a recently discovered photoreceptor in the eye. This may help those who don't respond well to traditional white-light therapy. Studies are under way to see if other types of light treatment, including synchronization to individual melatonin rhythms or simulated dawns, might improve individual health and performance.

New evidence from my laboratory—that it's not just our brains that make the powerful mood-enhancing beta endorphins in response to

UVB exposure but also our skin—is another major step forward. Most recently, my colleagues and I identified two genes in the skin that are responsible for regulating the body's circadian rhythms.

The discovery that we have biological clocks all over our bodies, not just in the hypothalamus, has also been a major breakthrough. These advances were initially made in research involving fruit flies and mice. Then, in a study that rocked the circadian rhythm research community, a group successfully reset people's body clocks by blindfolding them and exposing the area behind their knees to light. Although other research-ers have had difficulty replicating the results, this discovery has signifi-cant implications. It increases the likelihood that we may soon have the ability to treat a variety of other conditions associated with circadian rhythm disruption, including heart disease, diabetes, and even cancer.

The Dangers of Night Light

The profound impact that light can have on our bodies may also include an unwanted outcome, as new research links exposure to light *at night* to cancer. The association was first observed by Eva Schernhammer, M.D., who noticed that two of her colleagues—healthy women in their thirties—developed cancer with no risk factors or a history of the disease. Dr. Schernhammer worked rotating night shifts in a Vienna, Austria, can-cer ward from 1992 to 1999. She had to pull ten all-nighters a month in addition to her regular hours. When she landed at Harvard Medical School three years later, she curiously tapped into medical, work, and lifestyle records of nearly seventy-nine thousand nurses and discovered that nurses who'd worked thirty or more years on night shifts had a 36 percent higher rate of breast cancer than those who'd worked only day shifts. She continued to uncover unsettling news, and by late 2005 she published reports that her fellow female night owls exhibited a 48 percent rise in breast cancer. Blind women, on the other hand, had a 50 percent reduced risk of breast cancer, compared to their seeing counterparts.

These findings suggest that exposure to light at night may raise the risk of not only breast cancer but also several other types of cancer.

Future studies will bear this out. It also confirms the far-reaching influence that light can have on our bodies, notably our ability to fight diseases like cancer. It's not so much the light itself that is harmful, but rather what the light does to the body's physiology. Melatonin, it turns out, has powerful anticancer capabilities. All cells—including cancerous cells—have receptors that bind to melatonin, the hormone responsible for lulling us to sleep at night after the sun sets. When a melatonin molecule binds to a breast cancer cell, it counteracts estrogen's tendency to activate cell growth. Melatonin also affects reproductive hormones, which might explain why it appears to protect against cancers related to the reproductive cycle—ovarian, endometrial, breast, and testicular. Another feature of melatonin's cancer-fighting strength is its ability to boost the body's production of immune cells that specifically target cancer cells.

Dr. Schernhammer's studies, published in the *Journal of the National Cancer Institute* in 2001, provide the first evidence that there's a biological relationship between cancer and a disturbed circadian rhythm. This surely puts a new spin on the "graveyard" shift.

Sun, Brain Health, and Vitamin D

There's a reason I took a detour to cover circadian rhythm disorders that don't revolve primarily around vitamin D levels. The role sunlight plays in our biological clocks, which are directly tied to our physiological rhythms and thus, ultimately, to how we feel—sleepy or alert, hungry or full, hot or cold, and so on—reinforces the importance of sunlight in our lives. But now let's turn to how vitamin D plays directly into our mental health, starting with some interesting recent findings about vitamin D and dementia.

Dementia is among the most feared conditions of old age. No one wants to end up in a catatonic state characterized by the inability to communicate with others, recall memories, do simple math, recognize family members, and have a grasp on the goings-on in the world. Recently, two studies looked at the role of vitamin D in maintaining brain function. One examined evidence linking vitamin D deficiency to brain dysfunction, and the other explored the role of vitamin D in preventing the collapse of mental performance. Taken together, many of these reports lay the groundwork for the hypothesis that vitamin D can reduce the risk of dementia.

The term *dementia* is a bit misleading because it's not necessarily a single disease. Rather, dementia encompasses a spectrum of brain-related diseases, including Alzheimer's disease, vascular dementia, Lewy body disease, and what's known as frontotemporal dementia. The distinction between Alzheimer's, a progressive, degenerative disease of the brain that causes impaired memory, thinking, and behavior and is probably the most commonly thought-of brain disease of old age, and vascular dementia is somewhat blurred. As many as 45 percent of those with dementia may have mixed dementia, or a combination of Alzheimer's and vascular dementia. Vascular dementia is typically characterized by previous strokes, heart disease, hypertension, and diabetes.

The multifaceted nature of dementia means that there is no single, defined path to dementia—there are many, from inflammation and oxidative stress (otherwise known as free-radical damage) to small strokes and the death of neurons in the brain. And there are just as many risk factors or conditions that often precede dementia, including cardiovascular diseases, diabetes, depression, osteoporosis, and even dental cavities and periodontal disease. Not only do all of these increase the risk of dementia later in life, but notice that they are all associated with low levels of 25-vitamin D. The laboratory evidence includes several findings on the role of vitamin D in protecting the brain and reducing inflammation. People with Parkinson's and Alzheimer's, for example, have been found to have lower levels of 25-vitamin D.

It's not that boosting levels of 25-vitamin D will reverse or cure dementia (though I would strongly suggest that patients already diagnosed with dementia keep their 25-vitamin D levels in the healthy range); the goal here is to maintain adequate 25-vitamin D levels to *reduce the risk* of the pathways that lead to dementia—namely, the ones I just mentioned.

A study done by University of Manchester scientists in collaboration with colleagues from other European institutions compared the cognitive performance of more than three thousand men between the ages of forty and seventy-nine years at eight test centers. This study, published in the *Journal of Neurology, Neurosurgery, and Psychiatry*, wound up being quite remarkable because it was the first to look specifically at the relationship between vitamin D and cognitive performance (for example, how fast you can multiply two times two). In studying this large population sample, the researchers took into account potential interfering health and lifestyle factors, such as depression, education, and level of physical activity—all of which can affect mental ability in older adults. They found that the middle-aged and older men with the higher levels of 25-vitamin D showed the best mental agility. In fact, the men with higher levels of 25-vitamin D performed consistently better in a simple and sensitive neuropsychological test that documents an individual's attention and speed of information processing.

The most unexpected finding of the study was that increased vitamin D and faster information processing were more strongly associated in men over the age of sixty, although the biological reasons for this remain unclear. The scientists concluded that vitamin D appears to have extraordinarily positive effects on the brain. The study also raises the possibility that vitamin D could minimize aging-related declines in cognition. We don't know exactly how vitamin D and mental agility may be connected, but it wouldn't surprise me to see future studies demonstrate vitamin D's role in increasing certain hormonal activity or other biological reactions that ultimately protect neurons and that confer healthier brains.

It's common for people with dementia to suffer disturbances in circadian rhythm, too, because of the damage occurring to their brains. A vicious cycle often begins, with the dementia-induced circadian rhythm disturbances exacerbated by indoor confinement and lack of exercise, both of which contribute to circadian rhythm disorders. A person with dementia typically has problems sleeping through the night and may wander out of bed and be confused. Sedatives have traditionally been used to treat circadian rhythm symptoms associated with dementia, but they are not particularly effective and have significant side effects. A number of studies have proven that bright-light treatments can be extremely helpful. As you can deduce on your own by now, bright-light therapy helps people with various forms of dementia by resetting their biological clocks, helping them become more alert during the day so they go on fewer night wanderings. In addition, recent research has shown that reducing circadian rhythm disturbances using bright-light treatments can improve the mental function of people with early stages of dementia.

From Womb to Older Age

This brain protection actually beings in utero—in the womb. Living at higher latitudes has been shown to increase the risk of schizophrenia, the roots of which may take hold in a developing baby's brain long before symptoms emerge in young adulthood. In fact, one of the causal links that have been made between schizophrenia and vitamin D is based on the theory that vitamin D deficiency in utero alters brain development. This helps explain schizophrenia's odd characteristic of occurring more frequently in those born in winter or early spring. Dr. John McGrath, professor of pediatrics, biochemistry, and molecular biology at the Medical University of South Carolina, stated it perfectly when he said that vitamin D deficiency during pregnancy not only is linked to a mother's skeletal preservation and her baby's skeletal formation, but also is vital to the fetal "imprinting" that may affect chronic disease susceptibility later in life as well as soon after birth. That is to say, the vitamin D status of a pregnant woman directly impacts whether or not her child develops certain illnesses and diseases, from diabetes as an adolescent to osteoporosis and dementia as an elder.

To think that prebirth vitamin D determines our bone health for life and even our risk for cancer and autoimmune diseases, among a litany of other illnesses, is amazing. The connection wouldn't normally leap out at you, but the mounting evidence is clear and persuasive. Even a child's lungs are affected by a mother's vitamin D levels. Asthma, a common childhood problem, has been linked to vitamin D deficiency in mothers. When the journal *Clinical and Experimental Allergy* in 2009 published an article entitled "Childhood Asthma Is a Fat-Soluble Vita-min Deficiency Disease," laypeople and doctors alike took notice. The paper outlined a strong link between vitamin D and childhood asthma. (I'll be going into much more detail about pregnancy and vitamin D in chapter 10.)

Given this deluge of new information, it's no surprise that people often have more than one vitamin D–sensitive disease during their lives. The question you're likely asking yourself now is, how bad is your deficiency?

CHAPTER 7

Are You Deficient?

*A quick self-test to determine your
level of deficiency*

When the body aches for something it needs, it often has a way of telling us. When we're dehydrated, thirst signals from the brain encourage us to drink. The same goes for being fuel-deficient (hunger), sleep-deprived (drowsiness), and even faced with serious danger. The famous fight-or-flight stress response exemplifies how the body maintains its own brilliant survival system for life. All animals, in fact, survive by similar mechanisms that don't require a high IQ or a Ph.D., much less a complex brain that can ruminate over the past and worry about the future. But what about sensing a vitamin D deficiency? How do you *know*?

It's funny to think that, with the exception of humans, animals that rely on the sun for energy and vitamin D know instinctively to soak in those rays. They may not pass a driver's test or read health books, but at least they "know" what's good enough for their survival needs. It's well documented, for example, that lizards who are vitamin D deficient seek out UVB radiation just as they would water when thirsty. Humans, on the other hand, have this extraordinary capacity—thanks to the advanced brains that afford us the ability to critically analyze and judge to our hearts' content, whether that judgment turns out to be right or wrong—to talk ourselves into and out of anything, including the very things that could be healthy or unhealthy. Sometimes, though, it pays to act like a lizard.

By now, if you've been digesting the previous chapters and thinking about your geography and habits in the sun, you probably have a feeling you're vitamin D deficient to some degree. You may even have the urge to run out and buy a bottle of vitamin D supplements and call it a day. Unfortunately, you can't satisfy a body's need for more vitamin D with a quick trip to the market like you can satisfy hunger and thirst with quick access to food and water. A body that has been deprived of adequate supplies of vitamin D for a while requires a long-term commitment to restocking the system day by day and month by month, slowly building it back up over time. That's what part II will be about, as I take you through on a fail-proof plan to elevate your vitamin D levels back into healthful territory—and keep them there.

If you are vitamin D deficient or insufficient, then your vitamin D tank is empty and needs to be filled as quickly as possible. Sun exposure for only a few days and over-the-counter supplements in pill form usually aren't enough.

A good (and quick) prelude to part II, however, is getting some general sense of a potential deficiency and what you can do to get tested under a doctor's care for a real diagnosis. And that's exactly what this chapter is about.

Pop Quiz

How many of the following statements apply to you?

- ❑ I rarely go out in the sun.
- ❑ I wear sunblock and cover up my skin when I go out in the sun, especially during the summer months or when I'm outside in the middle of the day.
- ❑ My wardrobe typically covers most of my skin, including arms and legs.

❑ I live above 35 degrees latitude in the Northern Hemisphere (north of Atlanta and Los Angeles).

❑ I live below 35 degrees latitude in the Southern Hemisphere (south of Sydney, Australia, Santiago, Chile, or Buenos Aires, Argentina).

❑ I do not take a multivitamin along with a vitamin D supplement every day.

❑ I do not take a separate vitamin D supplement every day.

❑ I do not eat wild, oily fish (salmon, mackerel, herring, sardines, etc.) two to three days a week.

❑ I do not eat a lot of mushrooms.

❑ I drink fewer than ten glasses of fortified milk or orange juice a day.

❑ I am naturally dark skinned or am of African or Hispanic descent.

❑ I am older than sixty.

❑ I am younger than twenty.

❑ I am overweight and carry a considerable amount of extra fat.

❑ When I press firmly on my sternum (breastbone) with my thumb or forefinger, it hurts.

❑ When I press firmly on my shins, I feel pain.

❑ I feel like I have less energy and muscle strength than I should.

❑ I take antiseizure or AIDS medication.

❑ I take glucocorticoids (e.g., prednisone).

❑ I have celiac disease.

❑ I have intestinal disease.

❑ I have had gastric bypass surgery.

If you checked any of the above boxes, then there's a high chance that you suffer from a vitamin D deficiency. If you checked several boxes, then I encourage you to take part II's protocol seriously and, if you're curious, ask your doctor to test your vitamin D status. It's important, though, to make sure you request a specific test.

Testing, Testing, 1-2-3

The only surefire way to know for certain the extent of your vitamin D deficiency is to ask for a 25-hydroxyvitamin D test, also called a 25(OH) D test. Again, this is the circulating form of vitamin D that the liver generates and that then becomes activated by the kidneys. While it's intuitive to think you'd want to test for the body's "active form" rather than just a precursor, testing for the activated vitamin D (1,25-vitamin D) actually does not give an accurate portrayal of your vitamin D status. And here's the rub: many doctors order the wrong test, and when the results come back showing a normal level of activated vitamin D, they think everything is D-okay. You could, however, be suffering from a serious deficiency even though your activated levels appear normal—or even elevated. This may sound incomprehensible, but not once you understand a few facts about vitamin D's biology.

Any doctor can order the 25(OH)D test for you, but if they use the wrong coding when submitting the claim to the insurance company, they won't get reimbursed and you will wind up having to pay for the test. (The actual cost of vitamin D testing can vary significantly depending on the lab used and whether a large number of assays are being performed by an individual doctor's office or hospital. The assay cost can range from approximately $40 to $225 per test, so ask your health care provider. Medicare currently reimburses you for $40.) The code for vitamin D deficiency is 268.9, or if the doctor has a code for osteoporosis or for other related diseases for vitamin D deficiency, he or she may be able to use that. But 268.9 is for vitamin D deficiency, and using that can help minimize costs and maximize reimbursements. (Other codes of interest: osteomalacia = 268.2; osteoporosis = 733.00; osteopenia = 733.90.)

The active form of vitamin D circulates at one thousand times lower concentration than 25-vitamin D, which, when created by your body from a supplement, has a half-life in your circulation of two to three weeks. The 25-vitamin D made by your body in response to sunlight, however, lasts *twice* as long in the body. Half-life simply refers to the amount of time it takes the body to eliminate one half of the total amount of 25-vitamin D and 1,25-vitamin D in your blood. On the other hand, the active form of vitamin D has a half-life of only two to four hours, meaning that the concentration of active D in your bloodstream is reduced by half every two to four hours. As you become vitamin D deficient, the body immediately responds by increasing the production of parathyroid hormone, which tells your kidneys to activate vitamin D, which is why your activated vitamin D (1,25-vitamin D) levels are either normal or elevated when you are vitamin D deficient or insufficient.

How is that possible? And how can you be vitamin D deficient if the kidneys then crank out more activated D? My guess is that your target tissues, namely your intestines and bones, still can't get enough, even though your blood levels are normal. Serum calcium is usually normal in the vitamin D–deficient state. Most physicians also trip up on calcium levels. That is to say, if they measure calcium levels in the blood and see nothing off the mark, they automatically assume this translates to a corresponding normal vitamin D status. But in fact this isn't necessarily true. Neither calcium levels nor activated vitamin D levels in the blood can tell you whether or not you are vitamin D deficient. You must measure 25-vitamin D; do not accept any other marker no matter what your doctor tells you.

So, where should your 25-vitamin D levels be? The unit of measurement used for vitamin D is nanograms per milliliter, and most experts—myself included—agree that vitamin D *deficiency* is defined as 25-vitamin D of less than 20 nanograms per milliliter. Vitamin D *insufficiency* is between 21 and 29 nanograms per milliliter. And vitamin D *sufficiency* begins at 30 nanograms per milliliter. To obtain the full benefits of vitamin D for health, many experts recommend that blood levels be closer to 40 nanograms per milliliter. The reason for this is that higher levels have been associated with a decreased risk for cancer, heart disease, autoimmune disease, and so on. Vitamin D intoxication is typically not seen until blood levels are above 150 to 200 nanograms per milliliter; lifeguards, for example, are famous for touting levels of 25-vitamin D in the 100–nanograms-per-milliliter range, and you don't hear about them falling victim to vitamin D toxicity—principally because they're getting most of their D from the sun and it's impossible to get too much from this source. Similarly, tanners who use tanning beds once a week typically maintain levels in the 40– to 60–nanograms-per-milliliter range throughout the winter. If you rely on supplements for your vitamin D, it takes about a month to fall below 20 nanograms per milliliter if your regular supplementation goes on hiatus.

The assay for 25-vitamin D is now the most ordered assay in the United States.

Here's another way to look at it: for every 100 IU of vitamin D you ingest through, say, a supplement, your blood level of 25-vitamin D increases by 1 nanogram per milliliter. This is why both children and adults need to be on at least 1,000 IU of vitamin D a day when they have inadequate sun exposure to satisfy their body's vitamin D requirement. I personally take about 2,700 IU of vitamin D daily from supplements and milk (this is in addition to any vitamin D I get from sensible sun exposure), and my blood level is 50 nanograms per milliliter throughout the year.

Reading Different Assays

There are two main assays that test a person's vitamin D status, one of which is better than the other.

Liquid chromatography tandem mass spectrometry (I know, it's a mouthful usually abbreviated as just LCMSMS) is, in my opinion, the state-of-the-art, gold-standard assay that determines your blood levels of both 25-vitamin D_2 and 25-vitamin D_3. What you care about is the total 25-vitamin D, so you'd simply add up the results of this assay to arrive at your grand total. For example, if your results show 20 nanograms per milliliter of vitamin D_2 and 15 nanograms per milliliter of vitamin D_3, then your total vitamin D is 35 nanograms per milliliter. What makes this assay best is that it can differentiate between the two types of vitamin D. Remember, vitamin D_2 is available only as a pharmaceutical. So if you're being treated for a deficiency using pharmaceutical-grade D_2 but your blood level of D_2 does not go up, that indicates that your body is not absorbing vitamin D_2.

The other assay out there is a radioimmunoassay. It measures only your total 25-vitamin D and cannot distinguish between D_2 and D_3. If you don't have a choice in which assay is used and are stuck with the radioimmunoassay, it's still a reliable source that can suffice. If possible, however, request the LCMSMS assay for a more in-depth analysis.

Why Age, Place, and Race Matter

I've already covered how these circumstances factor into the vitamin D–deficiency equation, but let me remind you briefly.

Age. The older you are, the harder it is for your body to make vitamin D from sunlight, because the precursor of vitamin D in the body declines with age. That said, the skin has a large capacity to make ample vitamin D despite this physical decline in the "assembly line." Assuming there's a 50 percent to 70 percent reduction in the body's ability to make vitamin D by the age of seventy, all a seventy-year old would need to do to be able to make plenty of necessary vitamin D is expose more areas of skin (say, the arms and legs) three to four times a week. The seventy-year-old won't make what a twenty- to forty-year-old will in the sun (the equivalent of a 20,000 IU supplement), but the 3,000 to 5,000 IU he makes will suffice. Unfortunately, older people are especially receptive to the alarmist warnings about excessive sun exposure. The elderly often decrease their sun exposure at a time when they need more of it to be healthy. Studies I have participated in have shown that well over half of Americans age sixty-five and older are vitamin D deficient. If you are a senior citizen, you need to be much more concerned about the risk of fracturing a hip because you are vitamin D deficient than about the risk of getting wrinkles or skin cancer. Consider this alarming statistic: approximately three hundred thousand hip fractures will occur in elderly men and women this year; 20 percent of those people will die within a year, and 50 percent will never regain mobility and will have to move to a nursing home. Although you may have heard that before, it bears repeating.

Lifestyle. The more time you spend indoors during daylight hours, the less opportunity you have to make vitamin D. The lifestyles of most Americans, Europeans, and others in wealthy nations far above the equator typically entail long indoor days and a fixation on avoiding the sun's UV rays during any time spent outside. This explains why nearly sixty million American children and teens—that's 70 percent of the entire youth population—may have less than sufficient 25-vitamin D in their bloodstreams. One in seven teenagers is now walking around in a totally deficient state.

Geographical location. If you live in a place with relatively long winters, you get less sun over the course of the year because UVB rays cannot hit the surface of the earth at the ideal angle for making vitamin D in the skin during those winter months. The ozone layer absorbs most of the UBV trying to reach your skin. Also, if you live in a city with lots of D-defying ozone pollution, your risk increases.

Race. People with very dark skin, especially those of African descent, find it difficult to make vitamin D from limited sunlight, as their ancestors evolved in a part of the world where sunshine was available year-round. That this kind of skin is not efficient at converting the sun's radiation into vitamin D isn't an issue in Africa because there are unlimited amounts of sunshine on that continent. However, when people of African descent live at northern latitudes, they often become vitamin D deficient because their superprotective skin might not convert enough of the less UVB-containing sunlight into vitamin D. Studies I have participated in show that up to 80 percent of elderly African Americans (over the age of sixty-five) are vitamin D deficient. The Centers for Disease Control and Prevention recently reported that 42 percent of African American women of childbearing age (fifteen to forty-nine years old) throughout the entire United States are vitamin D deficient by the end of winter—a remarkable number. On average, 40 percent to 60 percent of African American adults are vitamin D deficient. African Americans are at increased risk of a variety of conditions associated with vitamin D deficiency, including type 2 diabetes and more aggressive forms of cancer in the breast and prostate. Americans of African descent are also more likely to have forms of high blood pressure (hypertension) and heart disease that are more resistant to drug treatment. It took millions of years for equatorial inhabitants to develop their skin type in response to their geography, and it will take millions more for evolution to catch up with those who have migrated elsewhere and who no longer need such a skin type to survive in UVB-deprived territories.

Culture. Certain cultures require that their women cover themselves entirely in heavy clothing that blocks out the sun. This may explain why studies done on people in sunny spots across the Middle East and India and have found widespread vitamin D deficiency. Men are not excluded from this fate because another factor is at work here: both men and women in these regions tend to avoid the sun in general because they don't want their naturally dark skin to get any darker.

Who Should Order the Test?

If you have symptoms that are consistent with vitamin D deficiency and you have been taking a vitamin D supplement over the last six months in the range of at least 1,000 or 2,000 IU per day, then it's in your best interest to get tested. People who have or are at higher risk for the following health concerns also should consider getting their 25-vitamin D levels tested if they are not taking an adequate amount of vitamin D as I prescribe in chapter 10:

- family history or personal history of cancer
- high blood pressure (hypertension)
- osteoporosis/osteopenia
- osteoarthritis
- autoimmune conditions (such as lupus, ankylosing spondylitis, multiple sclerosis, rheumatoid arthritis, Crohn's disease, type 1 diabetes)
- PCOS (polycystic ovarian syndrome)

- schizophrenia
- depression
- migraines
- epilepsy
- diabetes (either type 1 or type 2)
- fibromyalgia
- general aches and musculoskeletal pain in the body that have not been diagnosed
- low-back pain
- joint pain
- muscle weakness
- chronic fatigue syndrome
- poor nerve conduction
- poor balance

If you're on Medicare, the test should be totally covered. With health-care costs continually scrutinized, physicians are quick to cut back on expensive and unnecessary tests. The 25-vitamin D assay can be costly at some labs, and doctors who are not knowledgeable about the vitamin D–deficiency epidemic may view such a test as gratuitous and unnecessary. Some doctors still don't believe vitamin D deficiency can happen in their patients. That said, oftentimes when doctors find that just one of their patients is (surprisingly) deficient, they begin ordering 25-vitamin D tests on all of their patients. First, find out how much your 25-vitamin D test will cost, and if it seems unreasonable, ask your doctor where you can go and get tested. If you reach a dead end, call your health-care provider or find another doctor. Word about vitamin D deficiency is finally getting around, which is why the test for 25-vitamin D is the most ordered test in the United States today.

PART II

THREE STEPS TO REBUILDING YOUR VITAMIN D LEVELS

CHAPTER 8

Step 1: Let the Sunshine In

*Practicing sensible sun exposure
for optimal health*

We have just seen why we all need enough vitamin D in our bloodstreams to ensure the health of our bones and to help prevent a variety of deadly diseases, including cancer, diabetes, multiple sclerosis, and hypertension. I have also hinted throughout the discussion that there's no better way to obtain your supply of vitamin D than to literally let the sunshine into your life.

Of all the lessons learned in this book, this one may be the hardest medicine to swallow: giving yourself permission to expose your skin for a specific amount of time in the sun—without sun protection. How much should you allow? When? And, most relevant to the debate, *why* bother if you can just pop a pill?

Why: Sun and Supplements Aren't the Same

Let me start my discussion of why I call for sensible sun exposure in addition to supplementation with this: it's not easy to boost your vitamin D status into the healthy range of at least 30 nanograms per milliliter through supplementation alone. There is so much published literature now to demonstrate that even 1,000 IU a day will not raise your blood level above 30 nanograms per milliliter. Rachael Biancuzzo, my student, and my group just published a study of mostly healthy adults living in

Boston during the wintertime showing that 1,000 IU vitamin D_2 or vitamin D_3 a day did not raise their blood level above 30 nanograms per milliliter.

I liken this phenomenon to the concept of The Real Thing. Which would you prefer: a cubic zirconia or a diamond, *the real thing*? A generic can of soda or a Coke, *the real thing*? A virtual trip to Hawaii at an IMAX theater to see the lava oozing from the volcanoes or an actual trip to view them in person on the Big Island, *the real thing*? I assume you'd choose the latter in all these decisions. Well, if the body could say which method it prefers to get its daily dose of vitamin D, it would hands down give a standing ovation to sunlight sources of vitamin D rather than a bottle. After all, why else would it spend so many millions of years perfecting this clever and self-regulating process? There's something to be said for the fact that the body can in no way overdose on vitamin D created through sunlight, as it can through supplementation. I think that fact alone speaks volumes about what we should be doing. Another way to look at it: if you were Mother Nature and wanted to guarantee that all vertebrates and humans got an essential vitamin hormone, what better way than from the sun?

Here's something else to consider: vitamin D made in the skin lasts at least twice as long in the blood as vitamin D ingested from the diet. When you are exposed to sunlight, you make not only vitamin D but also at least five and up to ten additional photoproducts that you would never get from dietary sources or from a supplement. So the obvious question is, why would Mother Nature be making all of these vitamin D photoproducts if they weren't having a biological effect? My colleagues and I are in the process of identifying the photoproducts to see if they have a special biological function. In the meantime, we're going to expose men with prostate cancer to simulated sunlight using a specific sunlamp called the Sperti lamp (www.sperti.com) to raise their blood level of 25-vitamin D to the same level as that of patients who are taking oral vitamin D_3 (from Vital Nutrients of Middletown, Connecticut) and see whether there is some additional benefit.

And then there's the straightforward fact that sunlight is freely accessible. It doesn't ask for money in exchange for its dose of health, and it can impart more than just the raw ingredients to make vitamin D in the body. Sunlight, as we've seen, boosts mood, keeps the circadian rhythm in check, and helps us sleep soundly at night so we can rejuvenate and rehabilitate the body before another day.

Our richest source of vitamin D is the sun. Most of us need only a few minutes a day of sun exposure during the summer months to maintain healthy vitamin D levels throughout the year.

How Much?

I want to be clear right from the get-go that I do not advocate tanning, and I recommend you get only enough sun exposure to establish and maintain healthy 25-vitamin D levels and to improve your psychological health as Mother Nature intended. At the same time, if you have decided that the feeling of well-being you get from UVB exposure far outweighs the dangers, I would not discourage you from UVB exposure in excess of that which is needed for good health, as long as you know and accept the risks and never burn.

Clearly, just because "some is good" doesn't mean that "a lot is better." Undesirable consequences can result if you get too much sun, just as if you eat or exercise too much. Those consequences include non-melanoma skin cancer and wrinkles. (I'll be addressing the skin-cancer-sun-melanoma issue head-on in this chapter, so hang tight.) If sun is essential for good health, but too much can be unhealthy, this raises an obvious question: what is the right amount? I have been at the forefront of developing a scientific answer to this question and providing easy-to-use guidelines for the public.

If I diagnose osteopenia, osteoporosis, or osteomalicia in someone whose blood test reveals she is vitamin D deficient (the 25-vitamin D in her blood is less than 30 nanograms per milliliter; 1/33,000 of a gram in 1 gram of blood), then I will prescribe an intensive program to restore her 25-vitamin D level, generally consisting of 50,000 IU of vitamin D_2

weekly for eight weeks. This high-dose protocol can only be prescribed by a doctor. The alternative is to take 3,000 to 4,000 IU of vitamin D_2 or vitamin D_3 a day for eight weeks (you can buy a 1,000 or 2,000 IU supplement from your pharmacy). Although the patient's 25-vitamin D level will go up quickly, the symptoms related to vitamin D deficiency may take several weeks or months to lessen and many months to resolve completely.

Sun exposure is just as effective a way to build a person's 25-vitamin D level. If you sunbathe in a bathing suit on the beach or in your backyard, you will have received a dose of between 10,000 and 25,000 IU of vitamin D when you have sunbathed long enough to be slightly pink twenty-four hours later (technically, this is called a minimal erythemal dose, or "1 MED"). I always discourage anyone from getting a burn and always encourage protection of their face. Spending *one quarter to one half* the amount of time in the sun that it takes you to get pink is the safest way to build your 25-vitamin D levels, and doing this three times a week will provide you with a weekly dose of vitamin D equivalent to ingesting about 20,000 to 30,000 IU. This amount of sun exposure is usually enough to correct a vitamin D deficiency. If you work during the day, an indoor-tanning facility can provide the same benefits (and yes, I'll be addressing this hotly debated topic in this chapter).

I have calculated that to make approximately 2,000 to 4,000 IU of vitamin D you need to expose your arms and legs (about 25 percent of your body) for between one fourth and one half the time it takes your skin to be pink from the sun twenty-four hours later. This calculation is based on my finding that exposing most of your skin in a bathing suit to 1 MED will cause an increase in vitamin D in your body equivalent to taking between 10,000 and 25,000 IU of vitamin D orally. But actually it is equal to taking 20,000 to 50,000 IU of vitamin D in a supplement, because the vitamin D you get from the sun lasts twice as long in your body. Again, I want to stress that I am not advocating that you actually get 1 MED. However, it is important to figure out, based on your skin type and 1 MED time, how long your sensible and healthful sun exposure time is.

The Body's Rule of Nines
It helps to think of your body's total surface area in terms of percentages: Face: 9%
Arms: 18%
Abdomen and chest: 18%
Back: 18%
Legs: 36%
Other: 1%   If you are concerned about wrinkles, there is plenty of opportunity to get your vitamin D by exposing large parts of your surface area to the sun minus your face. Exposing your arms and legs will often do the trick in just a few minutes.

I have developed two ways for you to get the right amount of sun exposure for good vitamin D health. One is a commonsense guideline that depends on knowing your tolerance for the sun (the Holick Solution for Sensible Sun, described step by step on page 177). The other relies on the wealth of available scientific data I have accumulated and incorporated into a specific, user-friendly series of tables (the Holick Sensible Sun Tables on pages 180 to 188).

Sunscreens almost completely prevent the body from making vitamin D from the sun. SPF8 reduces vitamin D production by about 90 percent, SPF15 reduces vitamin D production by 95 percent, and SPF30 reduces it by about 99 percent. Therefore, do not use any sunscreen during the time specified for sensible sun exposure, but do put on a broad-spectrum sunscreen after that time has expired. Use a sunscreen with a sun protection factor of at least 15 (it's preferable to use SPF30 because most people don't slather on enough to actually achieve the stated SPF from their lotion) so you can enjoy being outside and minimize the sun's potentially harmful effects.

UVB radiation from sunlight does not penetrate glass, so you cannot make vitamin D from sunshine that warms your skin through a window. UVA, on the other hand, can penetrate glass.

But before getting too far into the details of sensible sunning, let's tackle the issue of skin cancer and premature aging caused by the sun.

Skinography and Mythology

That everyone can see your skin is just one indication of how important it is. It is your body's largest organ and weighs about six pounds. Skin provides a protective covering for your entire body and protects you from sunlight, heat and cold, infections, toxins, and injury. Other important functions of the skin are that it regulates body temperature and retains water. And, of course, your skin helps you convert sunshine into vitamin D.

Your skin has two layers, the outer epidermis and the inner dermis. These two layers are quite different. The inner dermis layer contains blood vessels, lymph ducts, nerve fibers and nerve endings, and hair follicles. It also contains sweat and sebaceous glands, which produce sweat to keep you cool and an oily substance called sebum that helps prevent the skin from drying out. Sweat and sebum get to the skin's surface through tiny holes called pores.

The outer epidermis is thinner than the dermis and is made up of squamous cells (also known as keratinocytes). Beneath these squamous cells are fuller-shaped cells called basal cells. Basal cells are constantly dividing to rejuvenate the skin. They rise to the top of the epidermis, where they are programmed to die and become the dead outer layer of our skin, known as the stratum corneum. This outer layer acts like a mirror to reflect UVA and UVB away from the skin. Underneath and interspersed between the basal cells are melanocytes. Melanocytes produce melanin, a pigment that gives skin and hair their color. The more melanin you have in your skin, the darker it is. For example, people of African descent have more melanin in their skin than people of Norwegian descent. The importance of melanin is that it absorbs the ultraviolet radiation of the sun, thus protecting the skin cells against sunburn. Because dark-skinned people have evolved to live in sunny regions, those with darker skin produce melanin all the time, whereas light-skinned people mainly produce melanin only in response to sun exposure. As you're about to find out, however, everyone who produces melanin in their skin—which is everyone except very fair-skinned or freckled, red-haired persons—has a natural defense against the sun's radiation.

Sunburn versus Suntan

One of the most important jobs of the epidermis—especially in light-skinned people—is to adapt quickly to protect skin cells from the sun's radiation. The defense mechanism the skin uses against sunburn is what we call tanning, which is an ingenious process. In response to sun exposure, the melanocytes produce melanin that makes the skin darker. The production of more melanin is triggered through an increase in the activity of an enzyme called tyrosinase. Melanin protects the skin by absorbing UV radiation. Even short bursts of sun exposure will trigger the melanocytes to produce more melanin.

Dark-skinned people do not have more melanocytes, but their melanocytes are more active, which explains why their skin is always pigmented. It also explains why the risk of all forms of skin cancer is lower for dark-skinned people—the cells of their skin are always more protected from damaging UVB and UVA by the presence of melanin, which acts like an umbrella, shielding the cell's vulnerable DNA and proteins from UV damage due to sun exposure. Melanin actually migrates upward and, like an umbrella, shades the nucleus of the cell from damaging UV radiation.

Sunburn is quite different from a suntan. When you get a sunburn, your skin turns red and can sometimes blister and peel. This redness, known in scientific terms as erythema, is actually caused by increased blood flow to the skin. This begins approximately four hours after the sun exposure and reaches its peak between eight and twenty-four hours after exposure. Blood is being sent to the skin to attend to cells that have been damaged by the sun. When severely damaged squamous and basal cells cannot repair themselves, they "commit suicide" so they won't replicate in a mutated state and cause cancer (this results in peeling). This form of cell suicide is known as apoptosis, or programmed cell death.

Fear of skin cancer is one of the main reasons for the hysteria over sun exposure. As is the case with so many health axioms, the relationship between sunshine and cancer isn't as straightforward as most people think. There are a number of myths associated with what causes skin cancer.

Myths Exposed

Many myths are associated with skin cancer, thanks to the barrage of public misinformation on this topic. Here are some of them. (I've touched upon many of these already, but they bear repeating.)

Any and all sun exposure causes skin cancer. Because UVB exposure is the easiest way to increase levels of 25-vitamin D, which humans can't live without, this statement needs to be questioned. While it's true that UVB radiation from sunlight—especially chronic overexposure to sunlight—is thought to be one of the causes of nonmelanoma skin cancer, virtually all nonmelanoma skin cancers are treatable and curable when detected early, and sunlight is proven to have protective benefits over the more deadly internal cancers. The trade-off between the risk of basal-cell carcinoma, for example, and the risk of stage 4 breast cancer cannot be understated. And you'll hear me state this more than once: there is no data to suggest that sensible sun exposure increases the risk of nonmelanoma skin cancer.

Sun exposure is the main cause of melanoma. There is no scientific evidence that regular, moderate sun exposure causes melanoma. As the FDA observed after a 1995 conference on melanoma, the relationship between melanoma and sunlight is baffling. Melanoma is seen more often in people who do not receive regular, moderate sun exposure than in those who regularly spend time in the sun. Most melanomas also occur on parts of the body that receive little or no sun exposure. This suggests that genetics plays a much more important role in the development of skin cancer than does regular, moderate sun exposure. There is also evidence that UVB-protection-only sunscreens may distort the UVB/UVA ratio that penetrates into the skin, thus contributing to melanoma development. Remember, UVA penetrates much more deeply than UVB, bombarding melanocytes and immune cells. Sunburns as a child or young adult increase a person's risk of melanoma, especially in areas *least* exposed to sunlight. A possible explanation for this is that sunburns may damage some melanocytes. Normally, this would trigger the immune system to jump into action to attack and kill the defective melanocytes. (This is known as immuno-surveillance and is a very good thing for keeping defective cells in check so they don't lead to cancer.) However, if the immune system is also affected by excessive UVB or UVA exposure, this immuno-surveillance system can become compromised. It then may no longer identify damaged melanocytes, and a major mechanism for preventing out-of-control melanocytes from growing into a deadly cancer is all but lost.

We are in the midst of a skin cancer "epidemic." It is inaccurate to call the increasing incidence of skin cancer an epidemic. Skin cancer rates have been rising steadily since the early twentieth century. Skin cancer rates are going up solely because more people are excessively sunbathing. Although skin cancer rates have been rising steadily since the early twentieth century, it wasn't until the 1960s that a tanned skin was considered desirable. Present-day people actually spend less time outdoors than did our forebears, most of whom worked the land before the Industrial Revolution. Working outdoors throughout the year probably helped previous generations build a resistance to sunburn in the form of tanned skin.

More recently—especially in the 1970s and 1980s, when a severe sunburn was considered a prerequisite for an eventual summer tan—people have become more likely to get sunburned. Adding insult to injury, the use of UVB-protection-only sunscreens probably contributed to the rise of melanoma because they promoted massive exposure to deeply-penetrating UVA. There's one hundred to one thousand times more UVA than UVB in sunlight. What's more, it helps to bear in mind that nonmelanoma skin cancer has an extremely low death rate. In the United States, it claims about 1,200 lives a year.

If you get regular, moderate sun exposure, you have less chance of developing malignant melanoma. New research shows that melanoma is more prevalent in Europe and North America than in the equatorial latitudes, which again suggests that regular sun exposure may prevent melanoma. At the very least, moderate sun exposure will not increase the risk of melanoma.

There's no such thing as a safe tan. Tanned skin protects you against sunburn, thought to be the main cause of melanoma. Also, it's more dangerous to avoid sun exposure completely than it is to get regular, moderate sun exposure. If you avoid getting sunburned, the benefits of sun exposure will far outweigh the possible dangers. Independent scientific research has shown that if you live in a sunny climate, or if you live in a not-so-sunny climate but expose yourself to sun, then your increased production of vitamin D due to UVB radiation will help lower risk of a host of debilitating and fatal diseases. Colon, prostate, and breast cancer—which together claim more than 115,000 lives each year—can in some cases be prevented by regular, moderate sun exposure. People who get regular, moderate sun exposure are less likely to get a malignant melanoma than those who don't. And don't forget about all the research backing sunlight's effect on a multitude of common illnesses and diseases, including internal cancers.

Tanning is like smoking to your skin. Wrong. Tanning is natural. It is your body's natural defense against sunburn. Smoking is an unnatural habit that your body rejects by becoming ill.

So What Is Skin Cancer?

Our bodies function normally when the cells that make up the different tissues—such as the prostate, breast, and colon—grow, divide, and replace themselves in an orderly fashion. Occasionally, cells divide too rapidly and multiply out of control; this can lead to cancer. Skin cancer results when this process occurs in the cells of the skin. There are several forms of skin cancer, but all of them fit into two broad categories: nonmelanoma skin cancer and melanoma.

Nonmelanoma Skin Cancer. By far the most common forms of nonmelanoma skin cancer are basal-cell carcinoma and squamous cell carcinoma (*carcinoma* is the medical term for cancer). Basal-cell carcinoma (BCC) affects the basal cells in the epidermis and is the most common form of nonmelanoma skin cancer. BCC usually occurs on areas of your skin that are most exposed to the sun and that are most likely to have been sunburned, such as the nose, face, tops of the ears, and backs of the hands. Often BCC appears as a small, raised bump that has a smooth, "pearly" appearance. Sometimes BCC looks like a scar and feels firm when you press on it. BCC may expand in size and spread to tissues around it, but these cells rarely spread to other parts of the body.

Squamous cell carcinoma (SCC) also occurs on areas of the epidermis that are most often exposed to excessive amounts of sun. Often SCC appears as a firm, red bump. The tumor may feel dry, itchy, and scaly, may bleed, or may develop a crust. SCC very occasionally spreads to nearby lymph nodes (lymph nodes produce and store infection- and cancer-fighting immune cells). SCC may also appear on parts of your skin that have been burned, exposed to chemicals, or had X-ray therapy.

Both types of nonmelanoma skin cancer are thought to be caused by long-term exposure to sunshine. Such exposure over many years may cause damage to the skin cells themselves so that they eventually start replicating out of control. Sun exposure over many years may also desensitize the skin's immune system in such a way that it will not recognize and act against cancerous skin cells.

Finally, researchers have been looking at the p53 gene, a "quality-control" gene that is responsible for fixing a damaged cell or causing it to kill itself (apoptosis). There is mounting evidence that the p53 gene system may be damaged by excessive, long-term sun exposure. Each person has two p53 genes—one from each parent. When one p53 gene is damaged, the skin cell becomes sick and multiplies abnormally to form a precancerous, scaly lesion known as an actinic keratosis. When both p53 genes are damaged and can no longer function properly, the skin cell may start replicating out of control and become a nonmelanoma skin cancer. The p53 gene is so important that it was declared the molecule of the year by the editors of the journal *Science* and appeared on the cover of *Newsweek*.

The likelihood that you will develop nonmelanoma skin cancer is greater if your exposure to sunshine began when you were a child, adolescent, or young adult. During these early years, the skin is especially vulnerable to sunburning. There is also the simple fact that the earlier in life that skin cells are damaged, the longer the chance they have to replicate in a mutated state. There's also more time to damage that second p53 gene.

Remember, not everyone who is exposed to strong sunshine from a young age is going to develop nonmelanoma skin cancer. Some people are genetically predisposed to this disease. This explains why certain people get nonmelanoma skin cancer while others don't—even when they have the same skin type and are exposed to just about the same amount of sun. It's also believed that a fatty diet may predispose you to a variety of cancers, including nonmelanoma skin cancer. People who suffer from DNA-repair-enzyme diseases such as a xeroderma pigmentosum (XP) also experience a much higher risk of skin cancer. XP is an extremely rare skin disorder whose sufferers are highly sensitive to sun exposure. The cause of XP is hypersensitivity of the skin cells to UV radiation due to a defect in the gene's DNA repair system. People with XP experience premature aging of the skin and multiple skin cancers. The disease is usually diagnosed in infancy when the child with XP exhibits severe skin problems, including skin reddening, scaling, and freckling. Skin cancers usually appear in early childhood, as do chronic eye problems. There is no cure for this disease, and the only course of action is to stay out of the sun.

Melanoma. Melanoma is a different story. Although rare, melanoma is much more deadly than nonmelanoma skin cancer. Comprising less than 5 percent of all skin cancers, melanomas are responsible for the majority of skin-cancer deaths, killing about 8,600 Americans annually. The number of new cases of melanoma in the United States has not changed much in the last eight years. Overall, the lifetime risk of getting melanoma is about one in fifty for whites, one in one thousand for blacks, and one in two hundred for Hispanics.

Melanomas occur in the deeper pigment-producing cells located between the dermis and epidermis, known as the melanocytes. When melanocytes become cancerous, or malignant, these cells grow uncontrollably and aggressively invade surrounding healthy tissues. Melanoma may stay in the skin, but more often it spreads, or metastasizes, through the blood or lymph system to the bones and organs, including the brain, lungs, and liver. Melanoma sometimes occurs in an existing mole or other skin blemish such as a dysplastic nevus (pronounced dis-PLAS-tik NEE-vus), but it often develops in otherwise unmarked skin. In men, melanoma develops most often on the upper back, and in women it is usually seen on the legs, although it may occur anywhere.

Melanoma is most common in people with fair skin and those who have a large number of moles, although it affects people of all races. Melanoma usually resembles a flat brown or black mole with an irregular, uneven border. Usually the blemish is not symmetrical. Melanoma lesions are often 6 millimeters (0.24 inches) or more in diameter. Any change in the shape, size, or color of a mole may indicate melanoma. A melanoma may be lumpy or rounded, change color, become crusty, ooze, or bleed.

There are numerous risk factors for melanoma. Excessive exposure to the sun is but one. But as you already know, melanomas occur in people who don't spend time in the sun and are often seen on parts of the body that aren't much exposed to the sun. Some of the nonradiation risk factors include the following:

- Heredity. If two or more of your family members have had a melanoma, you are much more likely to get one.

- Dysplastic nevi. These kinds of moles are more likely than normal moles to become melanomas.
- Many normal moles. If you have more than fifty moles on your body, this increases your chance of developing a melanoma because melanoma usually begins in the melanocytes of a normal mole.
- Weakened immune system. People whose immune system is weakened by certain other forms of cancer, certain drugs (such as cyclosporine) prescribed after organ transplants, or AIDS have a greater risk of developing melanoma.
- Previous melanoma. People who have already had a melanoma are at a high risk of developing another.
- Defective DNA repair system. People with the extremely rare skin disorder xeroderma pigmentosum (XP), described above, tend to have a defective DNA repair system and are at a higher risk of melanoma.

This brings us to the relationship between sun exposure and melanoma. Normal sun exposure of the type that builds a tan doesn't seem to be responsible for melanoma. Numerous studies pioneered by Drs. Cedric and Frank Garland, and Dr. Ed Gorham show that people who work outside have a lower incidence of melanoma than do people who work inside. Despite the fact that the United States was for several centuries a rural, agriculture-based nation whose citizens were outdoors much of the time, melanoma was so rare then that separate statistics weren't kept on the disease until the 1950s.

So what's going on? Why are melanoma rates increasing rapidly and have been doing so at a rate of 2 percent per year for more than thirty years? The answer is surprising—it may be because people are exposed to sunshine less during their working hours. *Sunburns* are a risk factor for melanoma. Because people these days—young and old alike—work outside less and therefore get less regular sun exposure than did previous generations, they are at increased risk of getting sunburned rather than suntanned when they do go out in the sun.

Another explanation for the rise in melanoma may surprise you even more: the use of sunscreens starting in the 1950s. Before any of you heave your sunscreen into the trash, let me make the point that the type of sunscreen that probably contributed to the rise of melanoma is the kind that protected only against UVB radiation. As I detailed earlier, until the late 1990s, UVB-protection-only sunscreen was all that was available, and this had been the case since the 1940s. In the past few years, this type of sunscreen has been phased out in favor of sunscreens that protect against both UVB and UVA radiation.

Recall when I explained that sunscreen was first developed to enable people to avoid sunburn and thereby spend more time in the sun, either tanning or participating in outdoor recreation. Although these early sunscreens protected against the burning radiation of UVB, they did not protect against UVA radiation. At the time, UVA radiation was not thought to be harmful because it didn't cause the obvious symptoms of sunburn. The increase in melanoma may be partially due to the fact that by protecting people against UVB, UVB-only sunscreen use enabled people to receive massive doses of UVA, which penetrates deep into the epidermis and dermis to damage the melanocytes and cause immune tolerance. We now know that UVA is partially responsible for melanoma, and the cosmeceutical industry has introduced sunscreens that protect against both UVB and UVA radiation—so-called broad-spectrum sunscreens. You should always use broad-spectrum sunscreen when trying to prevent sunburn. Look for sunscreens that clearly state they protect against both UVA and UVB, because discrepancies still exist in the market. Be aware, too, that no sunscreen can fully protect you.

With all this in mind, it is important to repeat that melanoma usually occurs in parts of the body that are not exposed to the sun and is seen in people who do not spend much time in the sun, two factors that indicate that sun exposure may *not* be a risk factor for this serious disease.

Going Home

Research in the last few years alone has finally begun to unravel the mystery of why melanoma can be so invasive, radically efficient in spreading quickly, and remarkably potent. Unlike other cancer cells, which take time to spread and can be clumsy in doing so, melanoma does not have to learn how to reach distant tissues and organs to inflict harm.

Usually, the movement of cancerous cells from one place to another, a process known as metastasis, is a highly inefficient and multistep process that requires cancer cells to leap many hurdles. First, cells must invade a nearby tissue and find their way to the bloodstream or lymphatic system to hitch a ride to a distant site, where they then disembark to establish new colonies. Melanoma seems to have this journey down pat, like the flip of a switch, and now we know how. It turns out that as melanocytes morph into cancer cells, they immediately stir a dormant cellular process that lets them travel swiftly through the body.

Key to this awakening process is a gene called Slug. (If you're hearing echoes of the "Snail" gene I talked about earlier, you're right; this is just another genetic ingredient that controls cellular functions and has an ironic name.) Slug plays an important role in allowing melanocytes to travel around the developing human embryo in the womb. These melanocytes begin in the midbrain of a developing embryo and migrate to distant sites, including the skin, during the embryo's development. But the Slug gene is permanently turned off once the melanocytes arrive at their destination. In 2005 researchers discovered that when melanocytes become malignant, they reactivate Slug—turning the gene back on. This gives the cell an immediate ability to spread, especially to the brain. It aims to "go home"—back from whence it came. The gene literally commands the cell to return home, and it also gives the cancer cell a road map to do so. This is why melanoma can be so deadly. Its power to turn Slug back on gives melanoma a tremendous advantage in spreading throughout the body.

Skin Type, Cancer Risk, and Self-Exams

Because melanin pigment protects skin cells against the damaging effects of the sun, certain people have higher rates of skin cancer than others. People with fairer skin (less pigmented and less protected) have a higher rate of skin cancer than people with darker skin (more pigmented and more protected). Scientists have categorized skin into six different types based on melanin content.

What Skin Type Am I?	
If you don't know your skin type and, thus, your relative risk for skin cancer, refer to the following table.	
I always burn, never tan, and am fair, with red or blond hair and freckles (albinos, some redheads, and some Scandinavians and Celts).	I have **type 1 skin.**
I easily burn, hardly get tan, and am fair skinned (people of Northern European origin, Germans, and some Scandinavians and Celts).	I have **type 2 skin.**
I occasionally burn and gradually tan (people of Mediterranean and Middle East origin).	I have **type 3 skin.**
I rarely burn and always tan (people of East Asian origin and some Indians and Pakistanis).	I have **type 4 skin.**
I seldom burn, always tan, and have medium-to-dark skin (people of African origin, South East Asians, and some Indians and Pakistanis).	I have **type 5 skin.**
I never burn and tan darkly (people with "blueblack" skin, people of African origin, and dark-skinned Asians such as Tamils).	I have **type 6 skin.**

People with type 1 skin have the highest risk of skin cancer and people with type 6 skin the lowest risk. If you have type 1 or type 2 skin and were exposed to excessive amounts of sun as a child, adolescent, or adult—including several severe sunburns—you are in the highest risk group for skin cancer and should get screened. Some people never get tan, principally those who are very fair skinned or red haired and freckled; they have type 1 skin. The reason people with type 1 skin don't tan is that the melanocytes in their skin are unable to produce protective melanin pigment. Because their skin is unprotected against the sun's radiation, these people are highly susceptible to sun damage, including sunburn, and are therefore at the highest risk for skin cancer.

One of the characteristics of skin cancer is that, unlike all other cancers, it is visible. If everyone were vigilant about detecting skin cancer in its early stages through self-exams, the mortality rate for nonmelanoma skin cancer would go down to virtually zero. We know how to catch skin cancer in its early stages, which is the key to reducing its severity. So the key to early detection and treatment of skin cancer is very much in your hands. There's no need for panic or overreaction, but you need to be on the lookout and know what to look for.

Just as women should do regular breast self-exams, each person should periodically check his or her skin for early signs of skin cancer. How often you do this depends on your risk factors. If you or a close relative has a history of skin cancer, or if other risk factors apply to you— such as if you have fair skin, burn easily, and had a lot of sun exposure as a child—examine your skin once a month. Otherwise, once every six months is probably sufficient. Checking yourself every day is counterproductive because you may not notice subtle changes that could be signs of skin cancer.

A red flag for skin cancer is a change in your skin's appearance, such as a new growth or a sore that doesn't heal. Look for these warning signs that you might have a nonmelanoma skin cancer:

- a lump that is small, smooth, shiny, and "waxy" looking
- a lump that is firm and red
- a lump that bleeds or develops a crusty surface
- a flat, red area that is rough, dry, itchy, or scaly
- a scarlike growth that gradually gets larger

If you see any of these changes on your skin, consult your personal physician immediately to determine their cause.

What about signs of melanoma? This very rare but dangerous form of skin cancer generally begins as an irregular-shaped, flat blemish colored a mottled light brown to black. Melanomas are usually at least one quarter inch across. The blemish may crust on the surface and bleed.

Melanomas usually appear on the upper back, torso, belly button, backs of the legs, lower legs, head, or neck. They also can be detected in the genital areas. Seek medical attention for a mole that changes size, shape, or color; a new mole; or a mole that looks odd or unsightly or begins to grow. Remember that pain is not an indicator of a skin cancer. Until it progresses to quite an advanced stage, a skin cancer won't hurt or sting. This fact reinforces the need to see a doctor as soon as you have any legitimate suspicion.

The Warning Signs of Melanoma

An effective way to remember the warning signs of a melanoma is to use this ABCD checklist:

❑ A: Asymmetry: one half is unlike the other half

❑ B: Border irregular: scalloped or poorly circumscribed border

❑ C: Color varied from one area to another: shades of tan and brown; black; sometimes white, red, or blue

❑ D: Diameter larger than the diameter of a pencil eraser (6 millimeters)

If you examine your skin regularly, you will become familiar with what on your body is normal. If you find anything suspicious during the course of your examination, see your doctor right away. Remember, the earlier skin cancer is found, the more straightforward the treatment program is and the greater the chance for successful resolution. If a doctor thinks a growth looks suspicious, he or she will order a biopsy. In this simple office procedure, the patient is given a local anesthetic and all or some of the suspect tissue is removed and examined under a microscope.

If skin cancer is diagnosed, there are various options for treatment. The doctor's goal will be to totally remove or destroy the cancer while leaving as small a scar as possible. Types of surgery include cryosurgery (destruction by freezing with liquid nitrogen), laser surgery (using a laser beam to cut away or vaporize growths), and curettage and electrodesiccation (using a spoonlike blade to scoop out the growth, then destroying surrounding tissue with an electric needle). Occasionally, other treatments, such as radiation therapy or chemotherapy, may be used alone or in combination.

Precise treatment and follow-up for both nonmelanoma skin cancer and melanoma depends on a variety of factors, including the cancer's location and size; the risk of scarring; and the person's age, health, and medical history. All of this is too complex to comprehensively cover in this book. An excellent resource for information on skin-cancer treatment is the National Cancer Institute. You can access its Web site at www.cancer.gov/CancerInformation/CancerType/skin.

How to Look for Skin Cancer

A good time to do a self-exam is after a shower or bath. Examine yourself in a well-lit room using a full-length and a handheld mirror. If you don't own a full-length mirror, use a three-way mirror in a private, well-lit dressing room at a clothing store. Start by learning where your birthmarks, moles, and blemishes are and what they look like. Check for anything new—a change in the size, texture, or color of a mole, or a sore that won't heal. The following are some other tips:

- Check everywhere, including your on your back, in your bellybutton, between your buttocks, and on your genitals (remember, melanomas often occur in non-sun-exposed parts of your body).

- Examine the front and back of your body in the mirror, then raise your arms and look at the left and right sides.

- Bend your elbows and look carefully at your palms, the top and underside of your hands and forearms, and your upper arms.

- Look at the front and back of your legs.

- Sit and closely inspect your feet, including between your toes.

- Examine your face, neck, and scalp. If necessary, use a comb or blow dryer to move your hair so you can see better.

Age and Excess

The regrettable fact is that almost all the damage to your skin from the sun occurs in childhood and early adulthood. If you're older than thirty, most of the sun damage that may have contributed to your risk of nonmelanoma skin cancer and melanoma has already taken place. Still, you can reduce your risk of skin cancer to some extent by being judicious about how much sun exposure you get in the future. Although sun exposure and sunburn early in life don't mean you will necessarily get skin cancer, your chances are higher.

Therefore, from the age of thirty onward you should focus on early detection. It's also important to educate younger family members about the risks of skin damage from long-term sun exposure and intermittent sunburn. Explain to them how they can safely get the benefits of sun exposure, an easy formula explained below. Folks over age seventy need not worry about trying to prevent skin cancer by staying out of the sun. In people of this age who have spent a lot of time in the sun, the damage has almost certainly been done. In addition to vigilance in regard to skin-cancer detection, the concern among older people should be whether they are getting enough sun to achieve and maintain a healthy 25-vitamin D level. Older people are much more likely to die from a vitamin D deficiency–related hip fracture due to osteoporosis than from skin cancer.

If you are younger than thirty and have had a great deal of unprotected sun exposure in your life, you should avoid any more UV exposure than is necessary to maintain good health. It is especially important that you protect against sunburn and stay within the limits of my formula for sensible sun.

The Holick Solution for Sensible Sun: Estimate, Expose, Protect

It's the million-dollar question: how do you manage this fine balance between risk and reward—the risk of skin cancer and the rewards of

UVB exposure? Here's how to use the Holick Solution to get sensible amounts of sun exposure and make enough vitamin D for good health:

1. **Estimate** how long it takes in the particular conditions in which you will be sunning yourself for you to get a mild pinkness (known as one minimal erythemal dose, or 1 MED).

2. Then, without applying sunscreen, **expose** your arms and legs for about 25 percent to 50 percent of that length of time. I have calculated that that amount of sun exposure two to three days a week enables the body to make enough vitamin D to stay healthy.

3. After getting this amount of sun exposure, **protect** your skin by putting on a broad-spectrum sunscreen with an SPF of at least 15, and preferably use SPF30. This will prevent overexposure and lessen the risk of skin cancer and wrinkles. The more skin you expose to the sun, the more vitamin D you will make. If you are wearing a swimsuit, it will take you less time per session than 25 percent to 50 percent of 1 MED to make the minimum amount of vitamin D you need for good health. Remember, it doesn't matter which area of your body is exposed to the sun, so long as at least 25 percent is. I don't recommend exposing your face, which comprises only 9 percent of your body's total surface area anyhow. Follow the directions on the sunscreen label to make sure you use the correct amount. SPF refers to the length of time a particular product protects against skin reddening from UVB exposure compared to skin without protection. For example, if your skin takes twenty minutes to begin reddening without protection, applying an SPF15 sunscreen should prevent reddening fifteen times longer—about five hours (though it may take up to twenty-four hours after sun exposure for redness to become visible). To maintain the SPF protection, it is important to reapply sunscreen every four hours and always after swimming. To get the SPF advertised on the product label, an adult in a bathing suit typically needs to use fully one quarter of a four-ounce bottle of sunscreen to cover his or her body. Studies have consistently shown that people do not apply enough sunscreen, which means they are not getting the protection they think they are.

Here's an example of the Holick Solution in action. Say you live in New York and frequent the beaches of Long Island. If you have quite fair skin (type 2 skin) and estimate it would take you half an hour of sun exposure on the beach at midday in July to be pink twenty-four hours later (because you haven't spent much time in the sun lately), then you should spend five to ten minutes—and up to fifteen minutes—in the sun before putting on sunscreen. This should not cause you to burn. If you are wearing a bathing suit and are exposing 75 percent of your body to sunlight, then your time without sunscreen can be reduced two to threefold and then just two or five minutes and up to ten minutes. Why not make more vitamin D in less time and fewer exposures? If you are a dark-skinned African American and can spend hours and hours out in the sun on the beaches of Long Island before getting burned—if you get burned at all—then spend half an hour in the sun before putting on any sunscreen. For those in between these two skin types who get pink in one hour, fifteen to thirty minutes of sun exposure will suffice.

You don't need to spend time on the beach to make vitamin D. You can do it sitting outside or walking while on your lunch break. But you do need to have your skin exposed to direct sunlight between the hours of 10:00 A.M. and 3:00 P.M. You cannot make vitamin D in high latitudes during the winter months. However, if you live in the northeastern United States and follow this guideline between May and October, you will make enough vitamin D to last you through the winter. Vitamin D is stored in your body fat and released in the winter when you need it. (However, if you are obese, this process is much less efficient, as the body tenaciously holds onto the vitamin D.) If you don't get this amount of sunlight between May and October, then during the winter months consider alternate forms of vitamin D, such as pill supplements and indoor-tanning facilities (for guidelines on this, refer to page 193).

Always adjust your calculations depending on the situation. For example, if you are at the beach at ten in the morning or four in the afternoon, the sun is less strong, so you can spend longer in the sun without protection. (If you estimate that at that time, based on your experience, it would take an hour for you to get a 1 MED, then you can spend about fifteen to thirty minutes in the sun without any sunscreen on.) Remember, I do not advocate that you ever get a mild sunburn, but simply that you estimate how long it would take you to get a 1 MED and make your calculations of sensible sun time accordingly.

What if you live in a climate such as Florida where the sun shines all year round? The same principle applies. You should try to get a few minutes of sun exposure two to three times a week for a length of time that depends on your skin type (see box) and the time of year. Make sure you take advantage of prime time: between 10:00 A.M. and 3:00 P.M. Even though at 7:00 A.M. the sun in Florida appears to be strong enough during certain times of the year to make vitamin D, its rays are not UVB-rich enough at this hour to make ample vitamin D.

The Holick Sensible Sun Tables

The second accurate and convenient method you can use to determine how much sun you need is with tables I have created based on my research. These tables provide sensible sun time for different climatic locations and different skin types.

The most important things you need to know before you start is what skin type you have and what latitude category you are in. Use the descriptions in the box on page 173 to determine your skin type. For these tables, I have divided the world into four main climatic regions: tropical, subtropical, midlatitude, and high latitude. Refer to the map of the world (figure 6) or to the U.S. map (figure 7) to determine the region where you live or the regions where you will be getting sun exposure.

You can also use tables 1 through 5 to help you determine the region where you live and how much sun exposure is sensible for you based on your skin type and the region and time of year.

Expose 25 percent to 50 percent of your body's surface area to 25 percent to 50 percent of 1 MED two to three times per week at all times of the year when you can make vitamin D in your skin (refer to tables 1 through 5 starting on page 182).

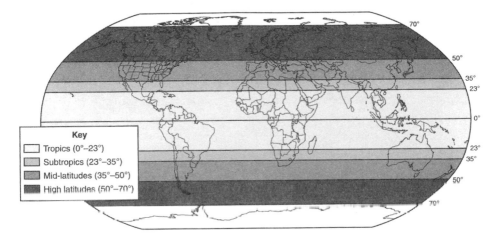

Figure 6. Map of the world broken down by regions of latitude.

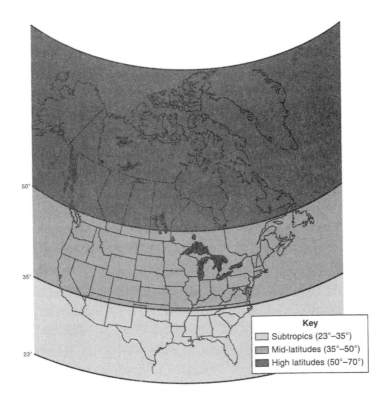

Figure 7. Map of North America broken down by regions of latitude.

Table 1. Latitude and Latitudinal Regions of U.S. and Canadian Cities

City	Latitude	Region
Albany, NY	42	Midlatitude
Albuquerque, NM	35	Subtropics
Amarillo, TX	35	Subtropics
Anchorage, AK	61	High latitude
Atlanta, GA	33	Subtropics
Austin, TX	30	Subtropics
Baker, OR	44	Midlatitude
Baltimore, MD	39	Midlatitude
Bangor, ME	44	Midlatitude
Birmingham, AL	33	Subtropics
Bismarck, ND	46	Midlatitude
Boise, ID	43	Midlatitude
Boston, MA	42	Midlatitude
Buffalo, NY	42	Midlatitude
Calgary, AB (Canada)	51	High latitude
Carlsbad, NM	32	Subtropics
Charleston, SC	32	Subtropics
Charleston, WV	38	Midlatitude
Charlotte, NC	35	Subtropics
Cheyenne, WY	41	Midlatitude
Chicago, IL	41	Midlatitude
Cincinnati, OH	39	Midlatitude
Cleveland, OH	41	Midlatitude
Columbia, SC	34	Subtropics
Columbus, OH	40	Midlatitude
Dallas, TX	32	Subtropics
Denver, CO	39	Midlatitude
Des Moines, IA	41	Midlatitude
Detroit, MI	42	Midlatitude
Dubuque, IA	42	Midlatitude
Duluth, MN	46	Midlatitude
Eastport, ME	44	Midlatitude
El Centro, CA	32	Subtropics
El Paso, TX	31	Subtropics

Eugene, OR	44	Midlatitude
Fargo, ND	46	Midlatitude
Flagstaff, AZ	35	Subtropics
Fort Worth, TX	32	Subtropics
Fresno, CA	36	Midlatitude
Grand Junction, CO	39	Midlatitude
Grand Rapids, MI	42	Midlatitude
Havre, MT	48	Midlatitude
Helena, MT	46	Midlatitude
Honolulu, HI	21	Tropics
Hot Springs, AR	34	Subtropics
Houston, TX	29	Subtropics
Idaho Falls, ID	43	Midlatitude
Indianapolis, IN	39	Midlatitude
Jackson, MS	32	Subtropics
Jacksonville, FL	30	Subtropics
Juneau, AK	58	High latitude
Kansas City, MO	39	Midlatitude
Key West, FL	24	Subtropics
Kingston, ON (Canada)	44	Midlatitude
Klamath Falls, OR	42	Midlatitude
Knoxville, TN	35	Subtropics
Las Vegas, NV	36	Midlatitude
Lewiston, ID	46	Midlatitude
Lincoln, NE	40	Midlatitude
London, ON (Canada)	43	Midlatitude
Los Angeles, CA	34	Subtropics
Louisville, KY	38	Midlatitude
Manchester, NH	43	Midlatitude
Memphis, TN	35	Subtropics
Miami, FL	25	Subtropics
Milwaukee, WI	43	Midlatitude
Minneapolis, MN	44	Midlatitude
Mobile, AL	30	Subtropics
Montgomery, AL	32	Subtropics
Montpelier, VT	44	Midlatitude

continued

City	Latitude	Region
Montreal, QC (Canada)	45	Midlatitude
Moose Jaw, SK (Canada)	50	Midlatitude
Nashville, TN	36	Midlatitude
Nelson, BC (Canada)	49	Midlatitude
Newark, NJ	40	Midlatitude
New Haven, CT	41	Midlatitude
New Orleans, LA	29	Subtropics
New York, NY	40	Midlatitude
Nome, AK	64	High latitude
Oakland, CA	37	Midlatitude
Oklahoma City, OK	35	Subtropics
Omaha, NE	41	Midlatitude
Ottawa, ON (Canada)	45	Midlatitude
Philadelphia, PA	39	Midlatitude
Phoenix, AZ	33	Subtropics
Pierre, SD	44	Midlatitude
Pittsburgh, PA	40	Midlatitude
Port Arthur, ON (Canada)	48	Midlatitude
Portland, ME	43	Midlatitude
Portland, OR	45	Midlatitude
Providence, RI	41	Midlatitude
Quebec, QC (Canada)	46	Midlatitude
Raleigh, NC	35	Subtropics
Reno, NV	39	Midlatitude
Richfield, UT	38	Midlatitude
Richmond, VA	37	Midlatitude
Sacramento, CA	38	Midlatitude
St. John, NB (Canada)	45	Midlatitude
St. Louis, MO	38	Midlatitude
Salt Lake City, UT	40	Midlatitude
San Antonio, TX	29	Subtropics
San Diego, CA	32	Subtropics
San Francisco, CA	37	Midlatitude
San Jose, CA	37	Midlatitude
San Juan, PR	18	Tropics
Santa Fe, NM	35	Subtropics

Savannah, GA	32	Subtropics
Seattle, WA	47	Midlatitude
Shreveport, LA	32	Subtropics
Sioux Falls, SD	43	Midlatitude
Sitka, AK	57	High latitude
Spokane, WA	47	Midlatitude
Springfield, IL	39	Midlatitude
Springfield, MA	42	Midlatitude
Springfield, MO	37	Midlatitude
Syracuse, NY	43	Midlatitude
Tampa, FL	27	Subtropics
Toledo, OH	41	Midlatitude
Toronto, ON (Canada)	43	Midlatitude
Tulsa, OK	36	Midlatitude
Victoria, BC (Canada)	48	Midlatitude
Virginia Beach, VA	36	Midlatitude
Washington, DC	38	Midlatitude
Wichita, KS	37	Midlatitude
Wilmington, NC	34	Subtropics
Winnipeg, MB (Canada)	49	Midlatitude

Table 2. Safe and Effective Sun Exposure (in Minutes) for Vitamin D Production: Tropical Latitudes (approx. 0–25 degrees, e.g., Honolulu, Jamaica, U.S. Virgin Islands)

Time of Year	Nov.–Feb.	Mar.–May	Jun.–Aug.	Sep.–Oct.
8:00 A.M.–11:00 A.M.				
Type 1 skin	10–15	5–10	3–5	5–10
Type 2 skin	15–20	10–15	5–10	10–15
Type 3 skin	20–30	15–20	10–15	15–20
Type 4 skin	30–45	20–30	15–20	20–30
Type 5–6 skin	45–60	30–45	20–30	30–45
11:00 A.M.–3:00 P.M.				
Type 1 skin	5–10	3–8	1–5	3–8
Type 2 skin	10–15	5–10	2–8	5–10

continued

Time of Year	Nov.–Feb.	Mar.–May	Jun.–Aug.	Sep.–Oct.
11:00 A.M.–3:00 P.M.				
Type 3 skin	15–20	10–15	5–10	10–15
Type 4 skin	20–30	15–20	10–15	15–20
Type 5–6 skin	30–45	20–30	15–20	20–30
3:00 P.M.–6:00 P.M.				
Type 1 skin	10–15	5–10	3–5	5–10
Type 2 skin	15–20	10–15	5–10	10–15
Type 3 skin	20–30	15–20	10–15	15–20
Type 4 skin	30–45	20–30	15–20	20–30
Type 5–6 skin	45–60	30–45	20–30	30–45

Table 3. Safe and Effective Sun Exposure (in Minutes) for Vitamin D Production: Subtropical Latitudes (approx. 25–35 degrees, e.g., Miami, San Diego, Los Angeles)

Time of Year	Nov.–Feb.	Mar.–May	Jun.–Aug.	Sep.–Oct.
8:00 A.M.–11:00 A.M.				
Type 1 skin	15–20	10–15	5–10	10–15
Type 2 skin	20–40	15–20	10–15	15–20
Type 3 skin	30–60	15–30	10–20	15–30
Type 4 skin	45–75	30–34	15–30	30–45
Type 5–6 skin	60–90	45–60	30–45	45–60
11:00 A.M.–3:00 P.M.				
Type 1 skin	10–15	5–10	1–5	5–10
Type 2 skin	15–30	10–20	5–10	10–20
Type 3 skin	20–30	15–25	10–15	15–25
Type 4 skin	30–45	20–30	15–20	20–30
Type 5–6 skin	40–60	30–40	20–30	30–40
3:00 P.M.–6:00 P.M.				
Type 1 skin	15–20	10–15	5–10	10–15
Type 2 skin	20–40	15–20	10–15	15–20
Type 3 skin	30–60	15–30	10–20	15–30
Type 4 skin	45–75	30–45	15–30	30–45
Type 5–6 skin	60–90	45–90	30–45	45–60

Table 4. Safe and Effective Sun Exposure (in Minutes) for Vitamin D Production: Midlatitudes (approx. 35–50 degrees, e.g., Hyannis, New York, San Francisco)

Time of Year	Nov.–Feb.	Mar.–May	Jun.–Aug.	Sep.–Oct.
8:00 A.M.–11:00 A.M.				
Type 1 skin	0	15–20	10–15	15–20
Type 2 skin	0	20–30	15–20	20–30
Type 3 skin	0	30–40	20–30	30–40
Type 4 skin	0	40–60	30–40	40–60
Type 5–6 skin	0	60–75	40–60	60–75
11:00 A.M.–3:00 P.M.				
Type 1 skin	0	10–15	2–8	10–15
Type 2 skin	0	15–20	5–10	15–20
Type 3 skin	0	30–40	15–20	30–40
Type 4 skin	0	30–40	20–25	30–40
Type 5–6 skin	0	40–60	25–35	40–60
3:00 P.M.–6:00 P.M.				
Type 1 skin	0	15–20	10–15	15–20
Type 2 skin	0	20–30	15–20	20–30
Type 3 skin	0	30–40	20–30	30–40
Type 4 skin	0	40–60	30–40	40–60
Type 5–6 skin	0	60–75	40–60	60–75

Table 5. Safe and Effective Sun Exposure (in Minutes) for Vitamin D Production: High Latitudes (approx. 50–75 degrees. e.g., Anchorage, Stockholm)

Time of Year	Oct.–Mar.	Apr.–May	Jun.–Aug.	Sep.
8:00 A.M.–11:00 A.M.				
Type 1 skin	0	20–25	15–20	20–25
Type 2 skin	0	25–40	20–30	25–40
Type 3 skin	0	30–50	25–40	30–50
Type 4 skin	0	45–60	30–50	45–60
Type 5–6 skin	0	60–90	50–60	60–90

continued

Time of Year	Oct.–Mar.	Apr.–May	Jun.–Aug.	Sep.
11:00 A.M.–3:00 P.M.				
Type 1 skin	0	10–20	5–10	10–20
Type 2 skin	0	15–25	10–15	15–25
Type 3 skin	0	20–30	15–20	20–30
Type 4 skin	0	30–40	20–30	30–40
Type 5–6 skin	0	40–60	30–40	40–60
3:00 P.M.–6:00 P.M.				
Type 1 skin	0	20–25	15–20	20–25
Type 2 skin	0	25–40	20–30	25–40
Type 3 skin	0	30–50	25–40	30–50
Type 4 skin	0	45–60	30–50	45–60
Type 5–6 skin	0	60–90	50–60	60–90

Are Tanning Beds Right for You?

In a perfect world, all of us would have the time and opportunity to strip off our clothes and step outside for several minutes a day for the amount of sun we need to make enough vitamin D to be healthy, especially between spring and fall, when we can stock up for the winter. Regrettably, that's not the case, and real life (not to mention office dress codes) tends to interfere with this goal.

Every day, approximately one million Americans frequent an indoor-tanning facility to look and feel better. Although I am not an advocate of tanning per se, I do believe in the importance of UVB exposure for making the vitamin D you need to be healthy and feel invigorated. If you don't have the opportunity to go out in the sun or prefer a more private and controlled environment, indoor-tanning facilities are a viable alternative to natural sunshine.

Am I crazy? Don't I know that tanning beds were officially listed as a carcinogen last year by the World Health Organization? And that the International Agency for Research on Cancer elevated sun beds to its highest cancer risk category? What kind of a doctor am I to be touting the benefits of sun beds when the powers that be have practically declared war on tanning salons?

I am a realist. I know that many of you will continue to frequent indoor-tanning facilities because of the way you look and feel afterward. I do understand the concern, though; tanning beds can be abused by people who don't know how to use them safely, especially the young, who are at high risk of damaging their skin for a lifetime. I also believe that if you have all the facts, you have the right to make the choice to enjoy UVB exposure indoors or outside. It's ludicrous and, frankly, irresponsible for the these institutions to say that tanning beds are on par with arsenic and mustard gas. Could the same be said about saturated fat and sodium? Certainly not. We need those for survival, just as we need UVB in moderation. And that's the message: moderation—a point I've been driving home since the first page of this book. So with all this in mind, if you choose to tan indoors, make sure you use this technology responsibly.

Thankfully, the indoor-tanning industry, through the efforts of the Indoor Tanning Association, is doing its part by introducing quality-control measures and offering education and certification for its personnel. Keep in mind that there's no such thing as artificial UV radiation. A UVB photon (packet of energy) is a photon whether it is produced by the sun or by a tanning bed with fluorescent lamps. The fact that the radiation you are exposed to in indoor-tanning facilities is the same as what you get from the sun means you need to take the same precautions you would if you were in the natural sunlight. As with natural sunlight, when using indoor tanning equipment there is the potential for the kind of overexposure that is associated with nonmelanoma skin cancer and prematurely aged skin.

Above all, make sure the indoor-tanning facility you use features appropriate equipment. At one time, indoor-tanning facilities used equipment that emitted high-intensity UVB radiation. When UVB radiation was linked to basal-cell and squamous cell skin cancer, the industry switched to UVA-only "high-pressure" lamps, which were considered safe because they didn't cause burning. Then it was discovered that UVA radiation may contribute to melanoma and wrinkles, as well as increase the risk of nonmelanoma skin cancer. Therefore, the trend in recent times has been toward low-pressure and medium-pressure lamps that emit a balance of UVA and UVB radiation (94 percent to 97.5 percent UVA and 2.5 percent to 6 percent UVB) that replicates natural sunshine. Before using an indoor-tanning facility, make sure it features low-pressure lamps (look for fluorescent tubes, not round lamps). Facilities that use high-pressure lamps should be avoided not only because of those lamps' potential for causing skin damage and certain types of cancers but also because they do not provide any sort of vitamin D benefit.

If you require assistance, find a facility where the staff has been certified by an industry association such as the International Smart Tan Network. A qualified staff member should do the following:

- Discuss your skin type and exposure-time charts carefully with you and ensure that you have access to this information at all times.

- Recommend an exposure schedule that will tan you moderately and avoid any pinkness and especially sunburn.

- Discuss with you anything that may cause you to react adversely to UV exposure (certain medicines, birth control pills, cosmetics, or soaps may increase your risk of a sun-sensitive reaction).

- Provide you with FDA-approved eyewear with usage instructions.

- Guide you through your first tanning experience.

Follow staff guidelines and those of the equipment manufacturers. Wear sun protection on your face. Do not exceed the recommended exposure time. Be aware that areas not usually exposed to sunlight can still get pink—another reason to consider spending less time than is recommended, which is supposed to be 0.75 MED. Indoor tanning exposure times are based on FDA and Federal Trade Commission guidelines, which allow a per-session UV exposure equivalent to 75 percent of 1 MED. This is quite liberal because you require only 25 percent to 50 percent of 1 MED (again, the time it would take you to get pink) to get enough vitamin D (equivalent to taking about 4,000 to 10,000 IU of vitamin D orally).

If you are concerned about the potential harm of UVB radiation and are not interested in a tan, you can get all the medical benefits of UVB exposure from just 25 percent of 1 MED (about 4,000 IU of vitamin D). One of the most popular reasons for using indoor-tanning facilities is to build a "base tan" in anticipation of a winter visit to a tropical destination such as the Caribbean. I think that's smart, and I'll explain why.

As I've made clear, I'm not a proponent of tanning, but I do believe in the importance of skin health and of protecting skin against strong sunshine. Increasing the melanin content in your skin by going to an indoor-tanning facility will provide you with a certain amount of natural protection against a burn. Start increasing the melanin content in your skin by visiting an indoor-tanning facility at least one month before you leave, and have three sessions a week. When you arrive at your tropical or subtropical destination, take the appropriate measures to protect yourself against a burn. Depending on your skin type, the protection you get from prevacation tanning salon exposure is equivalent to using a sunscreen with a sun protection factor of two or three (SPF2 or SPF3), which means you can stay outside two or three times longer than you could if you didn't have the "base tan."

Some people choose to purchase tanning equipment for use in their homes. I am in favor of doing this if your primary goal is to make vitamin D and improve your psychological health. Follow the same guidelines and precautions you would observe in commercial facilities or in natural sunshine. It is especially important to avoid overexposure, which can be a temptation because of your easy access to the equipment. Again, be sure your equipment uses low- or medium-pressure lamps—those that emit a balance of UVA and UVB radiation that most closely replicates natural sunlight.

Remember: Tanning beds that only emit UVA radiation will *not* produce any vitamin D in the skin. There's only one lamp on the market that has been approved to claim it helps boost vitamin D; you can learn more about the Sperti Sunlamp at www.sperti.com. My colleagues and I have shown that this lamp is very efficient in making vitamin D in the skin. Only three to five minutes of exposing the legs or abdomen three times a week can be effective. Dr. Vin Tangpricha, who spent time at Boston University and is now at Emory University running his own laboratory, and our group reported in 2007 that after only eight weeks of exposure, patients with cystic fibrosis who were unable to absorb vitamin D were able to significantly increase their 25-vitamin D levels.

Most people use tanning facilities for cosmetic reasons—in other words, to look and feel better. I use this kind of equipment extensively to test the effects of UV radiation on health. In one of the most dramatic examples of how indoor-tanning equipment can be used therapeutically, I managed to relieve excruciating bone pain in a woman with severe Crohn's disease who was vitamin D deficient because 90 percent of her intestines had been removed in surgery and no amount of oral vitamin D could enable her intestines to absorb enough vitamin D to keep her bones healthy. Her bone pain, caused by the condition known as osteomalacia (see chapter 3), was relieved in a month thanks to three-times-weekly sessions on a tanning bed, observing the manufacturer's exposure guidelines.

If you have trouble absorbing vitamin D from your diet, speak to your doctor about whether indoor tanning sessions would help correct your vitamin D deficiency. Three of the most common conditions associated with difficulty absorbing vitamin D through the small intestine are Crohn's disease, inflammatory bowel disease, and cystic fibrosis.

Lamps that emit UVB radiation were originally invented to treat medical conditions in the 1930s. Tanning beds as we know them today, however, didn't gain a foothold until much later. The man credited with being the "father of the tanning industry" is the Swiss engineer Friedrich Wolff. While studying the beneficial effects of ultraviolet light on athletes decades ago, Wolff took note of the tanned-skin side effect and went on to found the indoor tanning industry. Mimicking German and Eastern European spas, Wolff brought his European technology to the United States in 1978, and an industry was born to take advantage of people's desire to look as if they had just returned from an expensive vacation in the tropics. With the new information that vitamin D is so important for good health, I hope you will start to regard indoor-tanning facilities as places not to bronze yourself but rather to undergo therapy to stimulate your production of vitamin D. When my colleagues and I compared two groups of Bostonians—one a group of tanners and another who didn't tan, matched up in terms of age and sex, we showed that the tanners boasted a blood level of about 45 nanograms per milliliter, which, again, is thought to markedly reduce the risk of myriad health problems. Their counterparts who never visited a tanning facility, however, had 25-vitamin D levels in the 18-nanogram-per-milliliter range, far below the level required for maximum health protection.

Guidelines for Indoor Tanning

- Educate yourself. Know the pros and cons of UV exposure and how to use it and protect yourself.

- Use low-pressure or medium-pressure lamps. Look for beds that have fluorescent tubes, as opposed to round lamps. Ask the attendant working at the facility whether he or she knows for sure that the lamps at that facility are low pressure (those that emit a balance of UVA and UVB). High-pressure lamps emit only UVA, which penetrates deep into the skin and may cause skin cancer and wrinkles and alter your immune system. By definition, fluorescent tubes emit UVB, whereas round, high-pressure lamps emit UVA.

- Use common sense and practice moderation. Refer to the guidelines in this chapter for how much UV exposure you need. Keep in mind that indoor tanning facilities emit UV radiation equivalent to the sunshine at tropical latitudes. Restrict your exposure to 50 percent of the manufacturer's recommended time of exposure, or the time defined by my guidelines— whichever is less. Protect your face and wear lip sunscreen.

- Know the consequences of using oil. Rubbing oil into your skin flattens the very top layer of skin (the stratum corneum, which acts like a field of little mirrors reflecting the UVA and UVB) and increases the penetration of much of the UVA and UVB radiation that would otherwise be reflected off the skin. If you use such products, cut your UV exposure time by at least 30 percent.

- Wear goggles or peepers. Make sure the facility provides eyewear that fits snugly. If the facility offers goggles, make sure the goggles are sterilized after each use to prevent the spread of eye infections. If they are not, purchase your own pair of goggles.

- Consider your medical history. If you are being treated for lupus or tend to get cold sores, these conditions can be activated through exposure to UV radiation from indoor-tanning lamps, just as they are by natural sunlight. For example, if you carry the herpes virus, UV exposure to the areas affected, such as lips and the genital region, can induce activity of the virus and thus cold sores. Your skin may also be more sensitive to UV radiation if you take certain medications, such as antibiotics, antihistamines, tranquilizers, water pills, diuretics, or birth control pills. A well-run indoor tanning facility will keep a file with information about your medical history, medications, and treatments. Make sure you help the staff keep the file up to date.

Evolution and Adaptation at Work

We should give the human body more credit than it sometimes gets. People don't shrivel, shatter, or shut down at the first sign of stress. Instead, the human body operates on the "overload principle"—when subjected to outside forces, it adapts by getting stronger. Examples of this phenomenon abound in the human body.

Your muscles don't pop and your bones don't break if you regularly lift weights—they get bigger and more powerful so they can handle a heavier load. Your heart and lungs don't explode or collapse if you go running every morning—they become more efficient and your lung capacity expands. Your ligaments and tendons don't snap if you do stretching exercises—they get more flexible.

The same goes for your skin's exposure to sunshine. If your skin receives regular, moderate exposure to sunshine, it adapts by producing melanin to absorb the sun's radiation, thereby protecting itself against a future burn. It also induces DNA repair enzymes to spring into action. This is the human body's natural adaptation to outside stress. Of course, sudden and extreme exposure to strong sunshine after an extended period of nonexposure will result in sunburn in the same way that exposure to sudden and extreme physical activity can result in damage to the muscle-bone system or the heart.

Remember, too, that skin did not evolve solely to resist the power of the sunshine—your skin is also the conduit through which your body uses the sun's radiation to create the vitamin D you need for your very survival. Plus, you have an entire DNA-repair system made up of enzymes whose job is to repair damaged DNA and replace it with healthy new material. My colleagues and I are doing research to determine if the skin's DNA repair program is enhanced when it is exposed to moderate sunlight, and I suspect that it is. All this is to say that your body is designed to accommodate the effects of sunshine. To suggest that sunshine is necessarily harmful to your skin is to underestimate the human species' ability to adapt to its environment.

Antisun activists argue that to differentiate between the causes of nonmelanoma skin cancer and the causes of melanoma is to confuse the issue—they maintain that you need to avoid all sunshine and become a sunphobe. This ignores the fact that some sun exposure is necessary to survive and be healthy. The amount of sun exposure that causes the potentially deadly melanoma—an amount that results in a sunburn—should be stringently avoided, but the moderate, regular sun exposure, which is your main source of vitamin D and which is associated with the rarely deadly and easily treated nonmelanoma skin cancer, should not be forsaken. If it is, you increase your risk of developing a variety of more serious and deadly diseases.

Some people enjoy being in the sun and using indoor-tanning facilities so much that they will risk nonmelanoma skin cancer in favor of all the potential benefits of sun exposure. Others may choose to get only the minimum amount of UVB exposure necessary to build and maintain vitamin D levels. These are choices only you can make. However, we know a couple of things for sure. Subjecting yourself to unlimited amounts of UVB is potentially harmful. But denying yourself any and all UVB can lead to serious health problems if you are not taking enough vitamin D from dietary and supplemental sources to satisfy your body's requirement for vitamin D.

The Holick Solution for Sensible Sun is a guide to how much sun exposure you need to maintain appropriate vitamin D levels. Here's how it works. You estimate how long it would take for you to get a mild sunburn (when your skin gets pink—this amount of exposure is known as 1 MED), then two to three times a week, you expose 25 percent of your body (e.g., arms and legs) for 25 percent to 50 percent of that time. In other words, if it would take thirty minutes for your skin to get pink in the sunshine (as it would for me at noon on a Cape Cod beach in the summertime), then two to three times a week, spend eight to fifteen minutes in the sun before putting on SPF30 sunscreen. Use these guidelines if you choose to visit a tanning salon, too, but do not exceed 50 percent of the manufacturer's maximum recommended time of exposure.

CHAPTER 9

Step 2: Bone Up on Calcium

The dynamic duo of calcium and vitamin D
can sustain your life

Virtually everyone can recite the milk industry's campaign slogan: *It does a body good.* Much of this goodness no doubt hinges on the calcium content of milk. Calcium is the most abundant mineral in the human body, with over 99 percent of the amount present being found in the bones and teeth. For the growth and maintenance of healthy bones it is essential that we have sufficient calcium intake; we are at risk of developing bone diseases such as osteoporosis when calcium leaching is not balanced by dietary ingestion. But calcium is not only important for the skeleton; it also has a role to play in nerve function, blood clotting, muscle health, and other areas.

And, like an orphan child without a parent to guide it properly, calcium cannot work properly in the body without the help of vitamin D. Calcium and vitamin D share a special relationship that plays into everything about you, from your ability to build and maintain bone strength to your neuromuscular faculties and brain power. I've already touched upon these ideas in earlier chapters, but here I'll explore more about this calcium–vitamin D connection and encourage you to pay attention to your calcium intake as much as your vitamin D intake.

It is also well recognized that vitamin D aids in the absorption of calcium as well as phosphate.

The Missing Link Between Vitamin D and Bone Health

To discover that sunlight held a secret ingredient to preventing and treating bone diseases like rickets was one thing, but understanding why and how this all worked, from a single ray of UVB to health in the human body, was clearly another. It took scientists several decades to uncover the mechanism by which vitamin D produced in the skin could effect so many positive health benefits.

One of the reasons it took so long to tease out vitamin D's complex biological pathway and influence on other physiological processes is that we simply didn't have the tools to track vitamin D down. It wasn't until the mid 1960s that new laboratory techniques emerged to afford researchers the opportunity to follow vitamin D's intricate actions using radioactively labeled substances. Between 1969 and 1971, as I was making a name for myself in a renowned lab headed by Hector F. DeLuca at the University of Wisconsin, researchers, myself included, were making great strides in understanding the metabolic processing of vitamin D. By 1971 it was clear that vitamin D went through sequential transformations in the body that entailed inactive metabolites along the way until the kidneys converted the major circulating form (25-vitamin D) to activated vitamin D (1,25-vitamin D). These findings were confirmed by other teams of researchers, including Anthony W. Norman and his colleagues at the University of California at Riverside and Egon Kodicek and his coworkers at Cambridge University in England.

Isolating and determining the molecular structure of all these vitamin D metabolites helped put to rest the biggest mystery that had troubled vitamin D scientists for decades: just how did vitamin D influence calcium deposition to build strong bones? In the early 1950s, the Swedish researcher Arvid Carlsson discovered, much to everyone's surprise, that vitamin D can actually remove calcium from bones when it is needed by the body. At about the same time, the Norwegian biochemist Ragnar Nicolaysen, who had been testing different diets on animals for years, concluded that the uptake of calcium from food is guided by some unknown "endogenous factor." He believed this endogenous factor sent a message to the intestines that the body needed calcium. That message turned out to be activated vitamin D. With vitamin D's identity solved, answers began to emerge in the experiments tracing the activation of vitamin D.

Once we had our finger on activated vitamin D, and how it came to be in a complex series of conversions through organs and the bloodstream, it was apparent that we weren't dealing with just another vitamin. We were deciphering a previously vague and convoluted picture of how "vitamin D" worked on the body. And because of its profound effects, which we were just beginning to unravel and interpret, we quickly realized that it belonged in the hormone category. No sooner had we singled out 1,25-vitamin D, the active form of vitamin D, than we reclassified it as a hormone that controlled calcium metabolism, which refers to how the body maintains adequate levels of calcium (more on this below). This marked the genesis of understanding not only the relationship of vitamin D to the body's endocrine system and calcium regulation but also how vitamin D could effect positive change of myriad biological processes, from modulating the immune system to inhibiting the skin cell growth that leads to skin disorders like psoriasis.

As detailed in chapter 1, hormones are unique substances produced in the body. The word itself is derived from the Greek verb *hor man*, meaning "to stir things up." Acting as internal signals, hormones control not only different aspects of metabolism but also many other functions—from cell and tissue growth to blood sugar, heart rate, blood pressure, and even the activity of the reproductive system. By definition, hormones are produced by one organ and then transported in the bloodstream to a target organ, where they can cause a specific biological action. Evidence for reclassifying the active form of vitamin D came with the realization that 1,25-vitamin D is produced by the kidneys and that its secretion by the kidneys into the bloodstream, where it can then travel to the small intestine, leads to its buildup in cell nuclei of the intestine, where it regulates the efficiency of the absorption of dietary calcium. By 1975, Mark R. Haussler at the University of Arizona confirmed the discovery of a protein receptor that binds the active vitamin D metabolite in the nuclei of cells in the intestine.

With vitamin D now associated with the intestine, scientists were zeroing in on the mechanism of calcium control. It was noted that as the level of calcium in the diet rises, the amount of active vitamin D hormone in the body falls, and vice versa. This feedback-loop pattern further confirmed the idea that active vitamin D was a hormone, specifically a calcium-regulating one. The hunt was then on to find out how this exceptional hormone was linked to the rest of the body's endocrine system. My research colleagues and I found that a hormone produced by the parathyroid gland (hence called parathyroid hormone) is critical to maintaining adequate levels of active vitamin D hormone in the blood. When calcium is needed, the parathyroid gland sends this hormone to the kidneys to trigger production of vitamin D hormone. That hormone, in turn, prompts the intestines to transfer calcium from food to the blood. When calcium intake is too low to support normal functions, both vitamin D and the parathyroid hormone trigger a process in which stored calcium is mobilized from the bones (as Arvid Carlsson discovered fifty years ago). It does this by signaling bone-forming cells called osteoblasts to express on their surface a protein known as RANKL (receptor activator of NF-kappaB ligand), which acts as a magnet to attach to monocytic cells (a type of white blood cell) in the bone marrow. This intimate connection results in the birth of giant cells with multiple nuclei that release acids and enzymes to dissolve bone and unleash its stored calcium into the bloodstream.

Too often people discredit, or simply don't know, the role of calcium in their everyday functions. Calcium is required for skeletal and cardiac muscle contraction, blood-vessel expansion and contraction, secretion of hormones and enzymes, and transmission of impulses throughout the nervous system. The body strives to maintain constant concentrations of calcium in blood, muscle, tissues, and intercellular fluids, though less than 1 percent of total body calcium is needed to support these functions. The rest of your calcium—99 percent—is stored in your bones and teeth, where it supports their structure. And, as I explained earlier, bone itself undergoes continuous remodeling, with constant resorption (breakdown of old bone) and deposition of calcium into a newly formed bone collagen matrix. The balance between bone resorption and deposition changes with age. Bone formation exceeds resorption in growing children, whereas in early and middle adulthood the two processes are relatively equal. In aging adults, particularly among postmenopausal women and men over sixty years old, bone breakdown exceeds formation, resulting in bone loss that increases the risk of osteoporosis over time.

We all need calcium to survive, just as we need water. But there is a certain balance to be struck, a so-called homeostasis. In fact, you can think of the homeostasis of calcium ions in the body as a center of gravity for a number of physiological processes. If there is too little calcium in your blood (a condition called hypocalcemia), soft-tissue cells—especially nerves and muscle, which rely on calcium to operate— become dysfunctional. Your entire neuromuscular system will become abnormally excitable, and impulses may be triggered spontaneously. This, in effect, sends your body into convulsions as muscles, including those of the respiratory system, contract uncontrollably. In this situation, a person can die from failure to breathe. The heart, which also depends on calcium to beat properly, can lose its rhythm, with fatal consequences. Conversely, if there is too much calcium in the blood (a condition called hypercalcemia), organs calcify and eventually cease to work. This is especially true for the kidneys. Blood vessels will calcify, rendering them less pliant and thus increasing the risk of stroke and myocardial infarction. Those excess calcium ions have an opposite effect on the nervous system, abnormally depressing it and causing depression, constipation, and confusion. Having too much calcium can be just as hazardous as having too little.

So you can see how important it is to maintain steady and healthy levels of calcium in the body. You can also see how vitamin D promotes healthy bones by indirectly maintaining adequate serum calcium and phosphorus for bone mineralization to occur. Vitamin D controls the level of calcium in the blood. If there is not enough calcium in the diet, then it will be drawn from the bone. High levels of vitamin D (from the diet or from sunlight) will actually demineralize bone if sufficient calcium is not present.

We know that if you are vitamin D deficient, as most Americans are, your body will steal the calcium out of your bones. That is what would cause you to have osteopenia or osteoporosis, severe low bone density with increased risk of fracture. But being vitamin D deficient also prevents calcium from coming into the bones. And as a result, there's nothing more than a Jell-O-like collagen matrix left behind, and it will get hydrated just like Jell-O and water.

Women who complain of throbbing, aching bone pain are sometimes met with doctors who can't understand it. When the doctor presses on a patient's bones almost anywhere, she will often wince in pain, and that's because the doctor is pressing down where there's no mineralized bone on the surface. It's simply a Jell-O-like substance, triggering significant discomfort. The covering on the bone is full of nerve endings, and if there is no mineralized bone underneath it but instead a rubbery "Jell-O," then when the doctor presses on it, that compresses the covering and excites those nerve endings, resulting in pain. Like Jell-O, the collagen matrix expands under the periosteal bone covering, causing throbbing, aching bone pain. When people are sitting with aches in their hips or lying in bed with throbbing aches in their bones, it can be very hard for physicians to immediately think of vitamin D deficiency. But often that's exactly what's causing the problem.

Making sense of this remarkable relationship between calcium regulation and vitamin D has opened many new doors in science and medicine. In addition to shifting the course of treatment for people suffering from bone diseases, it has paved a new path for people suffering from calcium-regulation disorders due to underlying medical conditions. It suddenly became possible, for example, to treat patients who had lost their parathyroid glands or their kidneys and, as a result, could no longer regulate the level of calcium in their blood. Now that we had the ability to synthesize activated vitamin D hormone commercially, we could treat these patients with activated vitamin D and calcium. The effects were dramatic, putting an end to their painful muscle spasms, convulsions, and chronic bone disease.

Your Bones Savings Account

While calcium is a key mineral for both sexes, it is especially important to the health of women. After the age of thirty-five, most men and women start losing calcium from their bones due to poor calcium and vitamin D intake. During menopause, however, the rate of loss increases rapidly for women. It is therefore vital that calcium needs be satisfied through diet so that calcium is not leached from the bones. Maintaining sufficient levels during this period is critical if women are to avoid major skeletal problems. Not as well known is the fact that the degree of osteoporosis suffered in later life is largely dependent on the amount of bone mass achieved by early adulthood. For this reason, the building of strong bones—requiring regular calcium intake—should be a priority for women from childhood onward. By the age of eighty, 25 percent of men will have suffered a hip fracture. This is why men should be equally concerned about their bone health. Men have higher bone density than women because of higher muscle mass, but they, too, will lose bone mass. In fact, 12 percent of men will have an osteoporotic fracture in their lifetime.

When you are born, you are given a "bones savings account." This is where your body stores calcium. You are able to make deposits into this account for the first thirty to thirty-five years of your life. After that point, that account is in retirement, and whenever your body requires calcium, especially when it comes to remodeling bones, it can take from your dietary sources or it can take from your bones. Obviously, you want your bank account to be full and you want your body to use its savings as little as possible. You'd really like to have that account as an emergency fund and rely on your diet and supplementation to get the calcium you need. But if you end up with a measly account in midlife, your bones will pay the price.

Without an adequate, constant supply of calcium the bones become weaker and thinner and develop tiny holes or pores (a condition called porosity). These porous bones are what leads to osteoporosis. Currently ten million Americans—80 percent of whom are women—have osteoporosis. Moreover, thirty-four million Americans are considered to have bone loss that's a premature form of osteoporosis called osteopenia, which can progress to osteoporosis. Having either disease increases the risk of fractures in the hip, spine, wrist, pelvis, and ribs. Osteoporosis was once considered an older women's issue. However, as I've already pointed out, it can strike both sexes at any age and has been reported in children as young as twelve years old.

It is estimated that nearly 60 percent of dietary calcium is absorbed during childhood and adolescence, when bones are growing and need as much calcium as they can get. This is why teenagers are encouraged to ingest 1,300 milligrams of calcium a day. In adults the absorption rate decreases to 30 percent to 40 percent.

Luckily, calcium, unlike vitamin D, is easy to obtain from diet alone. Rich sources of calcium include dairy products (milk, yogurt, cheese), leafy green vegetables (including kale, escarole, collard greens, and bok choy), soy products (including tofu), nuts (especially almonds and pistachios), legumes, seeds, and calcium-fortified juices. Side note: although spinach is high in calcium, it's hard to get the calcium from it because it contains a lot of oxalate, a substance that tightly binds calcium so that it

How Much Calcium Do You Need Each Day?

Children	Calcium
1–3 years	500 mg/day
4–8 years	800 mg/day
9–18 years	1,300 mg/day
Adults	**Calcium**
19–50 years	1,000 mg/day
51 years and older	1,200 mg/day
Pregnant and Breastfeeding Women	
19 years or younger	1,300 mg/day
20 years or older	1,000 mg/day

cannot be absorbed into the body (not that spinach doesn't offer other nutritional benefits, however). If you eat well, then you may not need to take a calcium supplement. But if you feel that you're not getting enough (see box), then by all means add a calcium supplement to your daily regimen.

Soda Dilemmas

For several years now doctors have been debating the possible link between soda consumption and higher risk of osteoporosis. Does drinking lots of soda markedly increase your risk of bone disease by somehow toying with the body's calcium levels?

While it's been documented by several researchers that drinking soda is linked to osteoporosis, we don't understand exactly why this is the case. And while the phosphoric acid found in soda has been blamed for this correlation, it could be the simple fact that people (women especially) who drink lots of soda are not getting enough calcium from other beverages. That is, they are drinking calcium-devoid soda rather than calcium-rich milk or fortified juices to keep their calcium levels up.

One study, performed by researchers at Tufts University, looked at several thousand men and women and found that women who regularly drank cola-based sodas ("regularly" meaning three or more sodas a day) had almost 4 percent lower bone mineral density in the hip than those who didn't drink soda regularly. This was true even though researchers controlled for calcium and vitamin D intake. But women who drank noncola soft drinks, like Sprite or Mountain Dew, didn't appear to have lower bone density.

Clouding this study, however, and the issue at hand, are the potential effects of caffeine. We've long known that caffeine can interfere with calcium reabsorption in the kidneys, increasing calcium excretion into the urine. In the Tufts study, both caffeinated and noncaffeinated colas were associated with lower bone density. And the caffeinated drinks appeared to do more damage than the caffeine-free drinks.

The brouhaha over this debate will continue, but regardless, the "moderation" message should be obvious. Most people would do well to moderate their intake of these ingredients that, for whatever reason, seem to interfere with achieving ideal calcium levels in the body. When you limit soda and caffeine, you automatically move toward healthier ingredients overall that pack a more powerful punch of nutrition anyhow.

Calcium Supplements

Calcium supplements are an excellent alternative for people who fear their diet preferences are not giving them enough calcium. This is especially true for people who avoid dairy or who are lactose intolerant. The two main forms of calcium in supplements are carbonate and citrate. Calcium carbonate is more commonly available and is both inexpensive and convenient. The carbonate and citrate forms are similarly well absorbed, and both can be taken with or without food. One caveat, however, relates to people who don't make much stomach acid, as is the case for those taking a proton-pump inhibitor or hydrogen blocker (more on this coming right up). In this scenario, taking the calcium supplement with a meal is best. Other calcium forms in supplements or fortified foods include gluconate, lactate, and phosphate. Calcium citrate malate is a well-absorbed form of calcium found in some fortified juices.

How well your body absorbs calcium from a supplement depends, in part, on how concentrated elemental calcium is in that supplement. Absorption is highest in doses equal to or less than 500 milligrams. So, for example, if you like to take 1,000 milligrams of calcium per day from supplements, it's ideal to split the dose and take 500 milligrams at a time, two separate times during the day. Those who take a proton-pump inhibitor like Prilosec or Nexium to control acid reflux and gastroesophageal reflux disease (GERD), or Tagamet or Zantac (which work a different way but have the same effect of inhibiting the production of acid in the stomach), need to be extra careful about getting enough calcium. Because stomach acid helps the body absorb calcium by dissolving the calcium pill, thus freeing the calcium so it can be absorbed by the small intestine, lowering stomach acid levels may stop its proper absorption. In 2006, the *Journal of the American Medical Association* published a study suggesting that long-term (more than a year) use of proton-pump inhibitors in high doses increased the risk of hip fracture by 245 percent. The subjects in the study were all over the age of fifty, and the researchers said the effects were particularly exaggerated in people already at risk of osteoporosis.

However, if you take your calcium pill with a meal, as your meal is being ground up in the stomach so, too, is the calcium pill—without the need for stomach acid. This is why I tell my patients to take their calcium pill with their meals.

Some people who take calcium supplements experience gas, bloating, constipation, or a combination of these symptoms. These symptoms can often be resolved by spreading out the calcium dose throughout the day, taking the supplement with meals, or changing the brand of supplement used. The older you get, the harder it becomes to produce adequate stomach acid, as you did when you were younger (and able to down just about anything without gastrointestinal problems). For this reason, taking a calcium supplement with a meal is best.

Supplements that combine calcium *and* vitamin D are an even better option, as the vitamin, once it gets activated in the liver and kidneys, increases calcium absorption and provides other health benefits. Vitamin D is *essential* to the uptake of calcium from your diet, helping the calcium to become more easily absorbed in the bloodstream and bones.

Because of its ability to neutralize stomach acid, calcium carbonate is found in several over-the-counter antacid products, such as Tums and Rolaids. Thus these drugs serve two purposes—calming stomach acid and providing bioavailable calcium. The fact that you're chewing the calcium makes it easily absorbed.

People at Risk for Calcium Deficiency and Why
Postmenopausal women: Low estrogen stores dampen proper calcium metabolism and regulation.
Vegetarians: Avoiding diary and consuming mostly vegetables, some of which have compounds known to inhibit calcium absorption, including phytates and oxalate, act as a double whammy.
People whose diets include lots of protein and salt: High intake of sodium and protein increases calcium excretion.
Lactose-intolerant people: Those who have trouble digesting dairy products, and thus avoid them, are frequently found to be calcium deficient and have lower bone density.

The Diet Factor

Given the general state of our dietary habits, whereby processed foods take center stage in the lives of millions, I think a plausible argument to explain why many Americans fail to meet their calcium needs is the mere lack of good nutrition.

What's more, eating a healthy diet is a little-known but extremely important way to prevent skin cancer. A 1995 study published in the *International Journal of Cancer* reported that people who ate a low-fat diet had 90 percent less chance of getting skin cancer than those who ate a high-fat diet. Conversely, a diet high in fat shortens the time between UV exposure and the onset of skin cancer and increases the number of tumors that develop. According to this same article, the magnitude of the dietary effect is almost directly related to the amount and kind of fat consumed (saturated fat appears to be most closely related to skin cancer).

Unfortunately, for a century now, the American diet has been getting higher in fat—especially in the extra-unhealthy saturated fats. This may partly explain why skin cancer rates have gone up, as well as diabetes and heart disease. The average American diet is about 16 percent saturated fat, whereas most qualified dieticians will tell you it should be no more than one third of that. To make matters worse, there has been a trend toward fad weight-loss programs advocating high fat content (the Atkins diet is probably the best known of these).

Leaving aside whether these diets actually work in the long term to help people keep weight off, diets high in saturated fat may cause a variety of life-threatening health problems and probably contribute to skin cancer, not to mention all other types of cancer. But you don't necessarily have to go on a traditional "diet" to achieve the results you're looking for. You just need to start moving toward foods lower in saturated fat and try to limit or evict those foods that contain excessive amounts of fat—which is typically found in processed products (which also usually contain lots of salt and sugar) and marbled meats. There are several excellent eating plans out there that advocate eating this way.

It's beyond the scope of this book to offer specifics on the perfect diet, but I'll say that a healthy eating regimen calls for plenty of fresh fruits and vegetables, high-quality proteins ("high-quality" meaning they are low in saturated fat but can be high in healthy monounsaturated fats, as is the case with wild salmon), and whole grains.

The Benefits of Boosting Calcium: All the Way to Weight Loss

An estimated 44 percent to 87 percent of Americans don't get enough calcium, including children, who are falling severely short on this mineral critical for proper growth and development. Unfortunately, there are not usually any obvious symptoms of a calcium deficiency, and people can go for years in a calcium-deficient state before any noticeable problems occur. Most of the symptoms that might occur due to a calcium deficiency would be seen only if calcium levels are low in the blood. Because the body is very good at keeping the blood calcium levels steady (often at the expense of bone strength), most people will never experience any symptoms of a deficiency until their bones are significantly weakened and fracture.

The benefits of boosting calcium go far beyond the obvious reasons of helping to normalize calcium levels and ensure healthy physiological processing. Several recent studies have shown links between increased calcium intake and specific health benefits in an array of conditions.

Premenstrual syndrome. As noted earlier, Dr. Susan Thys-Jacobs of St. Luke's–Roosevelt Hospital Center in New York found a 50 percent decrease in PMS symptoms for women given calcium supplementation, compared to a 30 percent decrease for the placebo group. Thys-Jacobs concluded that "no other drug addresses all these symptoms as effectively." Another report, based on an epidemiological study of more than two thousand women, found a strong link between calcium and vitamin D intake and the risk of PMS. The authors concluded that "a high intake of calcium and vitamin D may reduce the risk of PMS."

Weight loss. Other studies at Creighton University, the University of Tennessee, and Purdue University have demonstrated links between increased calcium intake and weight loss. One of the researchers, Dr. Michael Zemel, reported that calcium plays a key role in metabolic disorders linked to obesity, and also that high calcium diets lead to the release of a hormone that leads to the body's fat cells losing weight. This is the basis on which the milk industry claims its product helps cinch a waistline, bolstering the "it does a body good" mantra.

High blood pressure. Clinical trials have also linked low calcium levels with high blood pressure. Argentinean research showed that women who take calcium during pregnancy may lower their children's future risk of blood-pressure problems. Studies done at Rockefeller University showed that calcium supplements were of general benefit to both mother and baby during pregnancy.

Colon cancer. Researchers at the University of North Carolina and Cornell University have linked calcium with the prevention of colon cancer.

Stroke. Harvard scientists reported on a link between increased calcium and the prevention of stroke.

Cholesterol. Researchers at the University of Texas Southwestern Medical Center have shown that increased calcium can lower LDL (bad) cholesterol.

The Ex Factor

You know you can't get through a health book without a mention of the "ex" factor, or exercise. I won't go into exhaustive detail about the benefits of exercise that you already know, if even subconsciously, by now. I won't even broach the subject of exercise's benefits in weight control, mood, cardiovascular health, and metabolism. But I will say that physical activity directly ties in to the conversation about bone and muscle health. Physical exercise, especially the weight-bearing kind, puts healthy stress on your bones to keep them strong and force them to be even stronger. It also works the muscles that keep you nimble and quick on your feet.

Young women and men who exercise regularly generally achieve greater peak bone mass than those who do not. Exercising allows us to maintain muscle strength, coordination, and balance, which in turn helps to prevent falls and related fractures. This is especially important for older adults and people who have been diagnosed with osteoporosis. The exercise you choose needn't be complicated, boring, or overly challenging or demanding. The best exercise for your bones is the kind that forces you to work against gravity, even if it's simply by working against your own body weight, as is the case for modern forms of yoga, mat Pilates, and the use of a resistance band. Other examples include weight training, hiking, jogging, climbing stairs, tennis, dancing, and, of course, walking. It's the constant pounding on the ground that translates to better muscle strength in the hips and lower back, maintaining or increasing bone density. These are the two places that are at highest risk for fracture.

So pick something you like and just go do it more often.

CHAPTER 10

Step 3: Supplement Safely

How to supplement as a backup plan

Whenever I give a presentation, one of the first things that happens is that all the attendees rush to their local pharmacy and buy a big bottle of vitamin D supplements. When they hear the story and appreciate what's going on, they get religion. (You can hear one of my presentations if you go to my Web site, www.drholicks dsolution.com.)

I was in South Africa, for example, giving some talks for a pharmaceutical company, and the president and CEO of the company was sitting in the audience. Immediately after my talk, he went out and got 1,000-IU tablets of vitamin D for himself and his family members. Once people hear the story and appreciate that there is no downside to increasing your vitamin D intake and there is a significant upside, everybody complies. But it's incomprehensible to many physicians that this simple vitamin that everybody has always taken for granted can have all of these health benefits. There is still great skepticism.

The driving force in convincing the medical community of the insidious consequences of the vitamin D deficiency epidemic has been mainstream media outlets, which promote the health benefits of vitamin D. This has included coverage in popular magazines and newspapers such as *Fitness*, *Vogue* and *Teen Vogue*, the *Wall Street Journal*, and even the *Enquirer*—both in print and on television in appearances by representatives of these publications. This has created a wave of awareness from the lay public to doctors, as media coverage of this information inspires viewers and readers to ask their doctors for a 25-vitamin D test. Some are met with hesitant, incredulous doctors. It's only after patients' insisting on the test that doctors reluctantly order it and likely find—much to their surprise—that their patients are vitamin D deficient. And testing from by doctors' offices of all of their patients commences.

My colleagues and I also find that if we can convince physicians to order 25-vitamin D assay on a couple of their patients, all the results come back as deficient. This often will convince the doctors. They've got religion, and now they order the test on all their patients. They realize that vitamin D deficiency is a major health issue. We've still got a long way to go in spreading this message about vitamin D, but those who are getting it really appreciate it.

Although I staunchly advocate that sunlight be most people's main source of vitamin D, vitamin D supplementation gets my seal of approval to make up for any shortfall in the vitamin D obtained from sensible sun exposure. Because you cannot overdose on vitamin D from sunlight, there's nothing wrong with taking a supplement to satisfy that "just-in-case" factor. Moreover, I know that there will be some people who just won't expose themselves to sunlight without protection. This choice may be based on personal fears, or it may be made in a unique case in which a person cannot go into sunlight for health-related reasons. People who take certain antibiotics or antihypertension medications that make them exceptionally sun sensitive, for instance, may opt to avoid the sun entirely and choose supplementation. Supplements may also be useful for people with type 1 skin, who have trouble going out into the sun without getting burned relatively quickly, and those with the rare disease xeroderma pigmentosum, who cannot expose their skin at all to the sun. Always remember that supplements are no remedy for poor nutritional habits, so it's important to eat a well-balanced diet. Otherwise, a nutritional supplement will be ineffective.

If you live at a high latitude but spend plenty of time outside during the summer months, then taking a vitamin D supplement during the winter may not be necessary, but it will make absolutely sure you have healthy 25-vitamin D levels year-round. To find out if you have enough 25-vitamin D, you can get your status checked with a blood test; at your request, your doctor will draw a small amount of your blood and send it off to a lab for testing (as explained earlier, make sure the doctor tests for your 25-vitamin D levels, not your levels of activated vitamin D, also known as 1,25-vitamin D). You want your 25-vitamin D levels to be in the range of 30 to 100 nanograms per milliliter of blood. Anything below 20 nanograms per milliliter is considered deficient, and anything between 21 and 29 nanograms per milliliter is insufficient.

Outdated Science, Inadequate Recommendations

In 1995, when the Institute of Medicine (IOM) formed an internal committee of which I became a member, we were asked by the National Academy of Sciences and the Food and Nutrition Board of the Institute of Medicine to make a recommendation on vitamin D intake based on published literature. We deliberated for two years. Dr. Robert Heaney, Dr. Bess Dawson-Hughes, Dr. Connie Weaver, Dr. Bonny Specker, and I were the experts in the field of calcium and vitamin D. We realized even back then, based on our own work that had yet not been published, that our recommendations were probably going to be inadequate; that is, although we knew from our unpublished investigations that the recommendations should be higher than what we suggested, we were obligated to make recommendations based only on published studies.

There was essentially none that was very relevant at that time. Most of the literature in the 1940s and 1950s showed that giving 100 IU of vitamin D to a child would prevent rickets, so doubling the dose to 200 IU was thought to be both effective and safe for preventing rickets in children. But rickets is the grossest manifestation of vitamin D deficiency; we now have a much more advanced knowledge about the effects of vitamin D deficiency far beyond rickets alone. Before 1997, when the IOM issued the new recommendations, the recommendation was 200 IU for everybody. In fact, it was determined by the Institute of Medicine in 1997 that there was insufficient evidence to establish *any* recommended daily allowance for vitamin D. Instead, a so-called adequate intake (AI)—a level of intake sufficient to maintain what was then perceived as a healthy blood level of 25-vitamin D—was established. The recommendations remain unchanged at this writing. The good news is that a new panel has been formed and plans to issue new recommendations this year.

We felt that we had made at least some contribution because we could, based on the literature published before 1995, show that at least 400 IU was needed to benefit adults ages fifty to sixty-nine, and 600 IU for people aged seventy and older. But now many experts agree that both children and adults need a minimum of 1,000 IU of vitamin D a day (and preferably 2,000 IU a day) to maintain a blood level of 25-vitamin D that we consider to be healthful, which is above 30 nanograms per milliliter.

It's a bit of a shame that even though all this fascinating and alarming research has emerged since 1997 to change our perspective on vitamin D, the government continues to advocate subadequate daily allowances. It takes time for such recommendations to formally change, though. I think that this year, with all of the emerging scientific studies being published in well-respected peer-reviewed journals, the newly formed IOM panel will suggest significant increases in vitamin D intake for children and adults. We've already watched groups within the medical industry, such as the American Academy of Pediatrics, publicly announce changes to their own recommendations in light of recent findings that call attention to the vitamin D deficiency pandemic and its consequences for infants and young children.

These scanty government recommendations are also holding back the food and multivitamin industry, as they continue to base fortification and supplementation levels on the Institute of Medicine's outdated recommendations regarding the safe upper limit, which is 1,000 IU for children up to one year and 2,000 IU for children older than one year and all adults. Most European countries still forbid the fortification of most foods with vitamin D. That's because of an observation in the

1950s, which turned out to be incorrect, that vitamin D intoxication in young children was due to the overfortification of milk with vitamin D. As a result of public outrage, European governments banned fortification of dairy products with vitamin D. They even went so far as to outlaw vitamin D in skin creams.

In my opinion, you could easily take 5,000 IU of vitamin D a day, probably forever. I typically recommend taking 1,000 to 2,000 IU of vitamin D a day—that should be adequate along with a multivitamin that contains 400 IU of vitamin D. I personally take 2,700 IU of vitamin D a day (400 in my multivitamin, another 2,000 from a stand-alone vitamin D supplement, and 300 from three glasses of milk). In the spring, summer, and fall, I cycle without sun protection for a period of time and then put sun protection on. We know from my own study, in collaboration with Dr. Robert Heaney, that you can take up to 10,000 IU of vitamin D a day for at least five months without toxicity.

You would have to take probably 30,000 to 50,000 IU of vitamin D a day for long periods of time, months or years, to become vitamin D intoxicated. The typical vitamin D intoxication incident is inadvertent, and usually, more than several hundred thousand IU to millions of IU have been ingested daily for a prolonged period of time. Vitamin D intoxication is one of the most rare medical conditions worldwide. You only need to be careful if you have a granulomatous disorder such as sarcoidosis, a rare autoimmune condition characterized by the formation of small lumps of cells ("granulomas"), usually in the lungs, where they can interfere with breathing, but sometimes in the skin, brain, and other organs.

How Much to Take and When

Of course, the major issue with obtaining vitamin D from a pill is that you have to remember to take the pill. Nowadays, it's easy to find supplements with 1,000 IU or even 2,000 IU per tablet or capsule. This wasn't the case just a few years ago. You can readily find supplements where you find other vitamins. Any national brand will do. There is even a liquid supplement from Wellesse that has 500 IU per teaspoon, which is ideal for children and adults who don't want to take a pill or have trouble swallowing pills.

Everyone from the age of one onward should be taking a 1,000 IU supplement daily in addition to a multivitamin that has 400 IU. In all, you will be ingesting between 1,500 and 2,000 IU of vitamin D daily among the supplements, multivitamin, and dietary sources. That's perfectly fine and right on target. (Don't forget to include calcium by drinking milk or orange juice containing calcium and vitamin D.) If your doctor tests you and determines that you are deficient, then you can certainly up the dosage to 5,000 to 6,000 IU a day under your doctor's care (again, this will be in addition to your multivitamin, so you'll be ingesting up to 6,400 IU a day for two to three months in supplement form). Depending on your level of deficiency, your doctor may prescribe a more aggressive treatment, with high doses of vitamin D for a certain time period. I treat with 50,000 IU of vitamin D_2 once a week for eight weeks (which is the equivalent of taking 6,000 IU a day) to fill an empty vitamin D tank. To maintain a full tank, I then administer 50,000 IU once every two weeks, which is the equivalent of 3,000 IU a day.

Remember, too, that it doesn't matter whether you take vitamin D_2 or D_3, though D_3 appears to be the most available form now on the market. (D_2 is the only form available as a pharmaceutical.) You also needn't worry about when or how to take it. Vitamin D supplements can be taken with food, with milk, or on an empty stomach. You do not need to ingest them with fatty food, contrary to a popular belief. I do suggest taking your vitamin D supplement when you take your multivitamin and any other supplements you might already be taking; get into the routine of taking this pill every day. Aging does not affect the body's ability to absorb vitamin D either from the diet or from supplements. And there is no advantage to taking smaller doses more frequently rather than one large dose of 1,000 to 2,000 IU a day. This also means that you could take either 1,000 IU of vitamin D once a day or seven 1,000 IU of vitamin D supplements once a week. It will work the same way, though I think this is an impractical way to go, as you are more likely to forget. If you forget just one day, you can take two pills the next day.

I recommend that everyone take at least 1,000 IU of vitamin D a day (and preferably 2,000 IU) along with a multivitamin containing 400 IU of vitamin D, all year long. This will not cause any buildup of vitamin D in the body, and by following this routine, you are less likely to forget it in the winter. For newborns in their first year of life, I recommend at least 400 IU a day and up to 1,000 IU. This is perfectly safe and may be more beneficial than just 400 IU (remember, Finnish children who took 2,000 IU a day for the first year of life had a 78 percent reduced risk of developing type 1 diabetes 31 years later). I recommend that children between one and twelve years old take at least 1,000 IU of vitamin D a day. For a breakdown of all my recommendations by age and condition, see the table on the following page.

Rectifying a vitamin D deficiency takes time. You won't see blood levels rise overnight. From my experience, healthy adults taking 1,000 IU of vitamin D a day can reach their peak blood level in five to six weeks. When I treat severely deficient patients with 50,000 IU of vitamin D_2 once a week for eight weeks, their blood level begins to increase by the first week and levels off by the fourth through sixth weeks of treatment.

For every 100 IU of vitamin D_2 or vitamin D_3 you ingest, you raise your blood level of 25-vitamin D by 1 nanogram per milliliter.

"Why Don't I Just Take a Supplement?"

That's the attitude of many people when they hear the new findings about the benefits of vitamin D. Their rationale is that by taking a vitamin D supplement, they can avoid the health risks of sun exposure while still availing themselves of all the health benefits of this vitamin. Unfortunately, it's not that straightforward.

For one thing, vitamin D taken orally—whether in whole foods or pill supplements—may not provide as much benefit as the vitamin D you get from the sun. The vitamin D you get from sunlight stays in your body longer and therefore provides longer-lasting benefits. In addition, sunlight causes your body to make not just vitamin D itself but also

How Much Vitamin D Should You Be Taking in Supplement Form?	
The following are my recommendations for adequate intake.	
0 to 1 year old:	400–1,000 IU per day (safe upper limit: 2,000 IU per day)
1 to 12 years old:	1,000–2,000 IU per day (safe upper limit: 5,000 IU per day)
13+ years old:	1,500–2,000 IU per day (safe upper limit: 10,000 IU per day)
Obese individuals:	2–3 times more than the above
Pregnant women:	1,400–2,000 IU per day (safe upper limit: 10,000 IU per day)
Lactating women*:	2,000–4,000 IU per day (safe upper limit: 10,000 IU per day)
*Lactating women who want to ensure their baby is getting enough vitamin D from their breast milk should take 4,000–6,000 IU a day.	

vitamin D–related substances called photoisomers. We are currently doing research on these photoisomers, which are made in the skin and could offer health benefits, but which are not present in supplements.

Keep in mind that neither vitamin D–rich foods nor supplements will cause your body to produce feel-good substances such as beta endorphins, which create the sense of well-being you feel after being in the sun or using an indoor-tanning facility. And nothing but the sun can regulate your circadian rhythm and maintain a healthy sleep-wake cycle.

Finally, unlike vitamin D supplements, neither sun exposure nor a tanning bed can cause vitamin D toxicity. Though difficult to do unless you're taking supplements that mistakenly contain toxic levels of vitamin D, if you overuse vitamin D supplements you are at risk of vitamin D toxicity. You cannot overdose by spending too much time in the sun or on a tanning bed. Vitamin D toxicity causes a number of serious symptoms, including nausea, vomiting, loss of appetite, constipation, increased thirst, increased frequency of urination, depression, and weight loss. Elevated calcium levels brought on by this condition can cause a variety of physical conditions, such as calcification of the kidneys, causing kidney failure, calcification of the major arteries, and confusion and bizarre behavior.

Vitamin D toxicity is defined as having levels of 25-vitamin D above 150 nanograms per milliliter with high blood calcium.

I don't mean this to alarm you, however. Vitamin D toxicity is extremely rare and happens only in unusual circumstances. My chief message here is the importance of both letting some sunshine into your life, as nature intended, and safeguarding your vitamin D levels by taking a supplement daily throughout the year. There is no harm in "doubling up" your vitamin D intake through sensible sun exposure and supplementation.

Double trouble: Do not double or triple up on your multivitamin to get more vitamin D. This can be dangerous because of other vitamins that you'd subsequently also be doubling or tripling up on and that can be toxic at high levels. Excessive amounts of vitamin A, for example, have been associated with birth defects and osteoporosis.

Supplementation During and After Pregnancy

The rules for pregnant women might surprise you. The IOM recommendation at this writing (200 IU of vitamin D a day) is inadequate for both pregnant and lactating women. My colleagues and I reported that 76 percent of pregnant women who took a prenatal vitamin (containing

400 IU of vitamin D) and drank two glasses of milk daily, thus getting 600 IU of vitamin D a day, were vitamin D deficient when they gave birth. And fully 81 percent of their newborns were vitamin D deficient. In my opinion, pregnant women need to be on at least 1,400 and up to 2,000 IU of vitamin D a day to maintain their blood level of 25-vitamin D above 30 nanograms per milliliter. A study currently under way suggests that a lactating woman can take as much as 4,000 to 6,000 IU of vitamin D per day without causing any toxicity either to herself or to her infant, and, more importantly, that it takes this amount of vitamin D to be transferred into her milk to satisfy the infant's requirement.

Human breast milk today contains little vitamin D today because lactating women take only 400 IU in a multivitamin and may get another 400 IU from a calcium + vitamin D supplement. This is a far cry from our hunter-gatherer foremothers, who were making several thousand IU of vitamin D a day that found its way into the milk to satisfy their infants' needs.

This is an ongoing study, and we do not know whether there are any long-term consequences for either the mother or the infant when the mother is ingesting 4,000 to 6,000 IU of vitamin D daily. From my experience, I would suspect that the study will show no toxicity and that it is perfectly safe to take this amount of vitamin D. Until the results come out, I will refrain from advocating that breastfeeding mothers take such a high dose of vitamin D, but I'd tell any new mother to at least increase her intake to 2,000 IU a day. Because most pregnant women take a prenatal vitamin, which will have 400 IU of vitamin D in it, adding another 1,000 IU to 2,000 IU in supplement form should be considered the bare minimum. This isn't about just the mother's health, but also that of her unborn child.

More than 50 percent of infants born in the United States are born in a vitamin D–deficient or insufficient state. As a consequence, they will not reach their fullest potential in height and bone density. Their condition can then worsen if they are not given enough vitamin D during infancy and childhood. One of the chief culprits here is the lack of vitamin D in human breast milk today, caused by lactating mothers' own vitamin D deficiency. It contains very little. Humans evolved to live much of their lives outdoors. For centuries people in agrarian societies spent hours outdoors, making thousands of units of vitamin D a day. Thus, this vitamin D could be stored in the milk for the infant's needs. Since the Industrial Revolution, our bodies haven't evolved to accommodate the shift to living mostly indoors, essentially evicting the sun from our lives.

As I outlined earlier, studies have linked vitamin D deficiency during pregnancy to an increased risk of the child's developing schizophrenia during his or her adult life. This goes to show how critical vitamin D is in the developing brain and psychological faculties of a fetus, even though we may not fully understand all the intricate mechanisms by which vitamin D helps safeguard the healthy development of a human very early in life. One thing is certain: vitamin D receptors are present in human embryos. And it's been shown that vitamin D deficiency during pregnancy is a risk factor for problems not only in fetal growth and calcium metabolism but also in the development of the fetal immune system. Don't forget that vitamin D also reduces the risk of pregnant women developing the serious complication preeclampsia. It also may make childbirth easier and reduce the need for a C-section.

Head sweating at night is one of the hallmark signs of vitamin D deficiency in a newborn.

Several studies have proved that women who take vitamin D during pregnancy also protect their young children from upper-respiratory-tract infections and wheezing diseases. Low levels of 25-vitamin D, in both mother and child, are also associated with a high risk of low birth weight and of the child's developing autoimmune diseases such as type 1 diabetes and asthma. Just recently, in the summer of 2009, a Finnish report published in the journal *Clinical and Experimental Allergy* stated that taking vitamin D during pregnancy was inversely associated with asthma and allergic rhinitis (inflammation of the nasal passages) in five-year-old children. That is to say, the women who took vitamin D during pregnancy were less likely to have children suffering from allergies and asthma by the time they were five years old.

Some experts have gone as far as making an association between vitamin D deficiency and autism, but there is no current proof that the two are related. We need more clinical trials to explore that connection further under the rigors of the scientific method. (However, there are vitamin D receptors in the brain, and vitamin D deficiency has been associated with poor muscle function; thus, it's important to ensure that children with autism have an adequate amount of vitamin D. Autistic children are often indoors, and vitamin D deficiency causes lethargy, muscle weakness, and a depressed mood.)

In chapter 2 I retold the dinosaur extinction story with a focus on vitamin D deficiency. I posited that pregnant females with a severe vitamin D deficiency would have had a difficult time producing viable egg hatchlings. Over time, the dwindling numbers of healthy dinosaurs able to procreate could have compounded other challenges they faced in a harsh environment that was no longer conducive to their survival.

Unlike the dinosaurs, humans—by virtue of our advanced brains and ability to develop technology—have managed to circumvent challenges posed by our circumstances, conditions, and in some cases our environment. (Though this last is increasingly the subject of debate over how our impact has altered the environment and whether we may someday face a fate similar to the dinosaurs'—no matter what technologies or brainy strategies we employ.) We've learned, for example, how to transport large amounts of clean water to distant, dry locations to sustain populations; we've mastered the art of agriculture and can fortify foods to boost nutrition. And we've developed ways to prolong human life and intervene with medicine when life-threatening situations arise, such as when a woman cannot give birth naturally for whatever reason.

Caesarean sections have been around since the Roman Empire, though the name mistakenly links them to Julius Caesar, who was not born by this surgical method of delivery. It used to be the delivery method of last resort when natural childbirth was not possible because of the health of or risks to the baby, the mother, or both. But in the last decade C-sections have gained popularity among women who prefer to schedule their deliveries (and not endure the pain of natural childbirth) rather than wait for their child to arrive vaginally after going into labor. Although the World Health Organization recommends that the rate of caesarean sections not exceed 15 percent in any country, the U.S. rate of births by C-section was 31.1 percent in 2006, the last year with available data.

This trend may reverse itself, however, as new studies point to other risks related to C-sections. Because C-sections are major surgery, they entail the usual additional related risks, from the use of anesthesia to respiratory difficulties and the need to stay longer in the hospital, where both the mother and child are at risk of developing a hospital-borne infection.

For women who plan on vaginal birth, the news that they need a C-section is not always welcome. They are not likely to be told that a vitamin D deficiency could be to blame, but it may just be.

In 2008, Anne Merewood and Dr. Howard Bauchner and my team reported a landmark study indicating that women who had low 25-vitamin D levels were more likely to have a C-section. The findings were part of a larger study that looked at the 25-vitamin D levels of women within seventy-two hours after delivery. None of the women in the study had previous C-sections, and the rate of C-sections in the study was 17 percent. We found 36 percent of these women to be vitamin D deficient and 23 percent to be severely deficient. We concluded that a woman with low 25-vitamin D levels is *four times* more likely to deliver by C-section than a woman with a higher level.

What's the connection? How can this be? Vitamin D doesn't have anything directly to do with giving birth, does it?

The reason behind this is actually quite straightforward, and you can think back to those dinosaurs for a moment to see why. Childbirth requires a certain level of strength to endure. A female trying to give live birth must undergo labor, which can last for hours or days. This trauma to a female's reproductive organs demands muscle strength and abdominal power. Granted, if females had to be athletes to give birth the human race wouldn't exist as we know it. Millions of women give birth every day who can hardly do a sit-up. But I'm not referring to just the obvious muscles employed during childbirth. The uterus itself is made of muscle, and as such, it can become weak and lose some of its strength if the person (or any vertebrate animal, for that matter, including a dinosaur) is overall vitamin D deficient. And if a woman's birthing muscles, including her uterus, are weak, this may hinder her ability to deliver the baby vaginally.

Clamping Down on Preeclampsia

One of the reasons a woman may find herself going in for an unplanned C-section is that she's been diagnosed with preeclampsia. It's among the most common yet more severe complications during pregnancy, a disorder characterized by sudden weight gain, fluid retention, high blood pressure, and swelling in the second and third trimesters. It can even last for a while after the woman has given birth. Other symptoms, including vision changes and headaches, may not always appear in rapidly advancing cases. Preeclampsia affects 5 percent to 8 percent of all pregnancies and is the cause of 15 percent of premature births. Preeclampsia is one of the most perplexing enigmas of pregnancy and has no cure; patients who suffer from it are monitored by their doctors to prevent further complications that threaten the life and health of both mother and child. Sometimes the condition can worsen to the point where a doctor will induce labor.

In collaboration with Dr. Lisa Bodnar at the University of Pittsburgh School of the Health Sciences, my colleagues and I reported that the occurrence of preeclampsia was *five times higher* in women whose 25-vitamin D measured low during early pregnancy. We also stressed that even slightly low 25-vitamin D measurements in pregnant women may double the likelihood of having the disorder. Even those who took prenatal vitamins showed a high risk for the deficiency. This isn't surprising given that prenatal vitamins don't contain enough vitamin D for proper supplementation.

Making Sure Your Baby Gets Enough

The American Academy of Pediatrics now recommends that all children, from birth through childhood, receive at least 400 IU of vitamin D each day. Most children can get this amount from drinking three to four servings of a vitamin D–fortified infant formula, milk, or orange juice, but infants who are breastfed exclusively will need an additional supplement of at least 400 IU. As I mentioned earlier, Wellesse makes a flavored liquid vitamin D supplement that can be mixed with infant formula, milk, or orange juice. It delivers 500 IU per teaspoon. You can also opt for a multivitamin that contains vitamin D in its mix. Speak with your pediatrician about which one to choose. Bear in mind that I believe 400 IU is the bare minimum and a total of 1,000 IU should be advocated.

Infants can be exposed to direct sunlight, but you should always protect their faces, as you would your own. At one year old, it's fine to graduate a child up to 1,500 IU vitamin D a day in supplement form. This can be in addition to fortified milk, infant formula, multivitamins, and sensible exposure to the sun. Trouble getting a child to swallow a tablet or capsule? Grind one up and mix it into a cup of milk or juice, or get yourself some liquid vitamin D from Wellesse or another manufacturer.

Putting the D in Diet

Though I've made it clear by now that it's virtually impossible to obtain an adequate amount of vitamin D from your diet, I must note that more fortified foods and beverages are likely to emerge on the market to help fill the gap. The top sources of vitamin D from diet are salmon (preferably wild), mushrooms, fortified orange juice and milk, fortified cereals, fortified bread, and fortified yogurt. Mushrooms may seem like an unlikely source for vitamin D, but not only do mushrooms naturally contain some vitamin D, growers are now exposing their product to ultraviolet light to enhance that vitamin D content. In collaboration with Coca-Cola, which owns Minute Maid, I did a study on the vitamin D content in their popular orange juice brand, showing that it was able to raise blood levels of 25-vitamin D in both children and adults. Below is a chart showing sources of vitamin D.

Source	Vitamin D Content
Salmon, fresh wild caught	~600–1,000 IU/3.5 oz vitamin D_3
Salmon, fresh farmed	~100–250 IU/3.5 oz vitamin D_3, vitamin D_2
Salmon, canned	~300–600 IU/3.5 oz vitamin D_3
Sardines, canned	~300 IU/3.5 oz vitamin D_3
Mackerel, canned	~250 IU/3.5 oz vitamin D_3
Tuna, canned	~236 IU/3.5 oz vitamin D_3
Cod liver oil	~400–1,000 IU/tsp vitamin D_3
Shiitake mushrooms, fresh*	~100 IU/3.5 oz vitamin D_2
Shiitake mushrooms, sun dried	~1,600 IU/3.5 oz vitamin D_2
Egg yolk	~20 IU/yolk vitamin D_3 or D_2
Sunlight/UVB radiation(i.e., UVB radiation from sunlight or a tanning bed with fluorescent tubes or a Sperti lamp).	20,000 IU equivalent to exposure to 1 minimal erythemal dose (MED) in a bathing suit. Thus, exposure of arms and legs to 0.5 MED is equivalent to ingesting ~3,000 IU vitamin D_3.
Fortified Foods	
Fortified milk	100 IU/8 oz usually vitamin D_3
Fortified orange juice	100 IU/8 oz vitamin D_3
Infant formulas	100 IU/8 oz vitamin D_3
Fortified yogurts	100 IU/8 oz usually vitamin D_3
Fortified butter	56 IU/3.5 oz usually vitamin D_3
Fortified margarine	429/3.5 oz usually vitamin D_3
Fortified cheeses	100 IU/3 oz usually vitamin D_3
Fortified breakfast cereals	~100 IU/serving usually vitamin D_3
Fortified bread	~100 IU/serving usually vitamin D_3

continued

Source	Vitamin D Content
Pharmaceutical and Supplemental Sources	
Vitamin D_2 (Ergocalciferol)	50,000 IU/capsule
Drisdol (vitamin D_2) liquid supplements	8,000 IU/cc
Multivitamin	400 IU vitamin D_2 or vitamin D_3
Vitamin D_3	400, 800, 1,000, and 2,000 IU

Note: Because of concern that vitamin D_2 is less effective than vitamin D_3, supplement and vitamin manufacturers have used the term vitamin D to represent vitamin D_2.

*Mushrooms are one of the only natural food sources that can provide different levels of vitamin D, depending on exposure to light. Mushroom growers can also enhance their products' vitamin D content by exposing them to more ultraviolet light. In general, shiitake mushrooms have the most vitamin D content (one cup of cooked shiitakes contains about 45 IU of vitamin D versus just 12 IU in a cup of cooked white mushrooms). Look for crimini (baby portabella) mushrooms in the grocery store that have been exposed to ultraviolet light, as they will also contain a high amount of vitamin D.

CHAPTER 11

Special Treatment

Other causes of vitamin D deficiency

N o day passes without hearing about another report on the obesity epidemic. No week goes by without a magazine rack displaying countless publications that shout out another trick to losing weight. Fast! Effortless! Fun! If it were that easy, we wouldn't see the obesity numbers continue to grow with our waistlines. Obesity-related conditions now account for nearly 10 percent of all medical spending, having doubled in the last decade. It's hard to believe that the obesity rate could rise 37 percent in just eight years alone, but that's exactly what happened between 1998 and 2006—bringing a breathtaking one third of the adult American population into the obese camp. Why the spike in such a short time frame? What really went on during those years that made it so incredibly easy (frankly, effortless) for millions—*millions*—of individuals to suddenly gain enough weight to qualify for this new and dangerous label?

Our bodies certainly didn't change, from an evolutionary standpoint. It's not like we woke up in the late nineties with bodies that could no longer metabolize food properly, but clearly we were doing something to tip the scales. Now, that whole discussion as to why and how this all occurred is a topic for another book. My point is that we now have a problem in our society so massive that it can no longer be considered *un*common. That is to say, obesity is a common health challenge today that gives rise to piles of other health challenges. And among these is vitamin D deficiency.

In this chapter, I'll share insights into underlying conditions that aggravate a vitamin D deficiency. Exposure to sunlight, diet, and supplementation aside, there are certain cases where keeping optimal levels of vitamin D is a serious uphill battle.

A Big, Fat Problem

Starting with the obesity issue is logical. It's colossal, affecting so many people as to be universal. It doesn't single out adults; rather, it's been reported that the current generation of American children may have shorter life expectancies than their parents because of the rapid rise in childhood obesity. The report, which was published in a 2005 *New England Journal of Medicine* piece, went as far as to say that childhood obesity could cut life spans by as much as five years. Clearly, it's not the obesity per se that's the killer—it's the associated diseases and complications: type 2 diabetes, heart disease, stroke, kidney failure, and cancer. The report also stated that the average life expectancy of adults, roughly seventy-seven years, has already been adjusted for the obesity epidemic. It's at least four to nine months shorter than it would be if there were no obesity. Obesity, it turns out, is already shortening average life spans by a greater rate than accidents, homicides, and suicides *combined*. We are, in effect, killing ourselves.

I described earlier how we've evolved to store vitamin D in fat. This allows us to have ample supplies on hand during the long winter months, when it's virtually impossible to make vitamin D—when the active synthesis of vitamin D from the sun is in hibernation until the spring. But humans did not evolve to carry such copious amounts of excessive fat that this fat begins to have negative effects on the body's metabolism and hormonal balance. Contrary to what you might think, overweight people don't have higher levels of 25-vitamin D due to their higher fat content. They have lower levels, because the excess fat absorbs and holds onto the vitamin D so that it cannot be used for bone building and cellular health. Unlike a normal-weight person, whose fat is continually being recycled so the vitamin D can be released, those with relatively immobile fat stores cannot access their vitamin D, which is literally locked up in their adipose tissue. Making matters worse, obese people are frequently vitamin D deficient to start with because they go outside much less, tripping a vicious cycle.

The price tag on obesity-related medical care is nearly 60 percent higher than expenses for all types of cancer combined.

It's been well documented by Dr. Norman Bell and by others, including my team, that obese people tend to have deplorable 25-vitamin D levels. Most obese people have muscle weakness and aches and pains in their bones and muscles and are lethargic. Vitamin D deficiency is associated with all of those symptoms. My team did a study to prove the point. We took obese and nonobese people and put them in tanning beds. Obese subjects raised their blood levels of vitamin D only 50 percent as much as normal-weight individuals. To be sure that this had nothing to do with body surface, we also gave an oral dose of 50,000 IU of vitamin D_2 to obese and to nonobese individuals and saw exactly the same phenomenon—vitamin D levels rose about 50 percent in the obese individuals compared to the nonobese individuals.

Clearly, the most effective treatment for these individuals is weight loss and higher doses of vitamin D to compensate for their impaired ability to keep up the 25-vitamin D level in their blood. Obese people need two to three times more vitamin D a day than those of normal weight, so I advise such patients to take between 3,000 and 6,000 IU of vitamin D a day. This does not entail any risk of toxicity and may even ultimately help a person to lose weight, given vitamin D's positive impact on insulin metabolism. It can also improve muscle strength, lessen aches and pains in bones, muscles, and joints, and inspire people to boost their activity level. The weight loss alone will likely have an impact on multiple medical levels, decreasing all the risk factors for vitamin D deficiency. As discussed earlier, the so-called metabolic syndrome typically seen in obese individuals is a collection of symptoms, including belly fat, which puts one at high risk of heart disease, stroke, and diabetes.

The heartbreaking truth about being obese, as anyone suffering from this can attest, is that losing weight is difficult. Genetics and environment aside, the mere condition adds another formidable obstacle to surmount. And some of that obstacle is linked to vitamin D and calcium. Studies have determined that sunlight, UVB, and vitamin D help normalize food intake and blood sugar. Therefore, weight normalization is associated with higher levels of vitamin D and adequate calcium.

When the diet lacks calcium, there is an increase in fatty acid synthase, an enzyme that converts calories into fat. Higher levels of calcium with adequate vitamin D inhibit this enzyme, while diets low in calcium increase this enzyme *by as much as fivefold*. More of this enzyme's activity means more fat getting stored from calories coming in. In one study, genetically obese rats lost 60 percent of their body fat in six weeks on a diet that had moderate calorie reduction but was high in calcium. All rats supplemented with calcium showed increased body temperature, indicating a shift from calorie storage to calorie *burning* (a process known as thermogenesis).

What this means is that in the presence of calcium and vitamin D, the body turns down the volume on this fat-storing enzyme. Without adequate calcium and vitamin D available, the body turns up the volume on this fat-storing enzyme, and what you end up with is just that—a higher volume of fat working against everything an individual would like to see happen in his or her body. This is yet another reason to focus on upping calcium and vitamin D intake while reducing caloric consumption to force the body to convert fat into fuel and reduce the weight load. As much as weight gain can feel like a spiral, so, too, can the weight-*loss* experience; as the pounds fall away, the domino effect of the benefits adds up and helps catapult the weight-loss efforts further. I've witnessed innumerable transformations among people who commit to losing weight and who consequently change their vitamin D status along the way. One of my patients who corrected a vitamin D deficiency lost thirteen pounds in six months, which for her was "those last ten pounds."

Obesity Surgery: A Cruel Paradox

In the summer of 2009, a surprising study emerged from the Mayo Clinic that the Associated Press posted with the headline "Obesity Surgery May Thin Bones, Causing Breaks. Bariatric Patients May Be More Likely to Fracture Hands or Feet."

It seems like a cruel joke. Why would obesity surgery lead to thinner bones? Wouldn't losing all that fat reverse the obesity-related problems, including vitamin D deficiency?

The irony in all this is that it turns out that obesity *protects* bones. Why? Because the body isn't stupid; obese people would crush themselves under their own weight if the body didn't increase its bone mineral density. What we don't know yet, though, is whether bariatric patients do end up with worse bones or simply go through a transition period as their bones adjust to their new body size. About fifteen million Americans are classified as extremely (morbidly) obese, defined as being one hundred pounds or more overweight. Diet and exercise alone don't help these people enough to stave off diabetes and other health problems, which is why surgery is fast becoming a popular option. There are currently two forms of the surgery, one that involves stomach stapling, called gastric bypass, and another that's less invasive, called stomach banding. Patients tend to lose between 15 percent and 25 percent of their original weight, and diabetes dramatically improves. More than 1.2 million U.S. patients have undergone the surgery in the past decade, 220,000 in the last year alone, according to the American Society for Metabolic and Bariatric Surgery.

We in the medical community have long known that radical weight loss can speed bone turnover, causing the breakdown of old bone to outpace the formation of new bone. Recent studies have shown that a year after gastric bypass, hip density among adult patients drops by as much as 10 percent. Stomach banding causes less thinning because it doesn't change as much how nutrients are absorbed into the body. We also know that gastric bypass makes it harder to absorb calcium, prompting doctors to advise their patients to increase their intake of calcium and vitamin D. Whether or not they comply is anyone's guess.

You would think that losing one hundred pounds of fat, with all the vitamin D in it, would boost 25-vitamin D levels, but my colleagues and I showed that it does not. The change in the transit time of food through the digestive tract adds another hurdle to the body's ability to absorb vitamin D from the diet. Likewise, other nutrients in the diet can be difficult to absorb.

Teams of researchers are currently trying to get to the bottom of this phenomenon and find out whether it translates into more fractures among gastric bypass patients. In one alarming observation, six years after surgery patients had more hand and foot fractures than a control group and had a nearly fourfold increase over their rate of such fractures before the surgery. Adding to the mystery is that the breakage was to the hands and feet, rather than other areas. Are these people getting more active in their lighter bodies and falling more as a result?

Because so many teenagers resort to this surgery—at a time when they are building their bone mass—there's a pressing need to examine the impact among adolescents and how they fare further down the road as a result of this surgery. One question yet to be answered: does gastric bypass surgery change the body's hormonal chemistry such that it can no longer support optimal bone strength?

Until now, bariatric surgery has called for annual screening of calcium, phosphorus, magnesium, and albumin (a blood protein). This new study, which underscores the increased risk of vitamin D deficiency among gastric bypass patients, calls for adding to this list both 25-vitamin D and parathyroid hormone, the chief hormones in calcium metabolism.

As with obese patients, I recommend that patients who have had gastric bypass surgery take two to five times as much vitamin D as a normal person—3,000 to 10,000 IU daily. To correct a deficiency, I have given patients as much as 50,000 IU of vitamin D_2 three times a week for eight to sixteen weeks to get their blood level of 25-vitamin D up to between 30 and 100 nanograms per milliliter. Then I put them on 50,000 IU of vitamin D_2 once or twice a week and monitor their serum 25-vitamin D level every one to two months until it stabilizes. One caveat: often these patients are unable to digest the gelatin capsule that the pharmaceutical vitamin D comes in, so I often advise them to cut the capsule open, put it into a glass of skim milk, swirl it around, and drink the milk without the capsule. I would implore all such patients to discuss this with their doctor. Maintaining healthy levels of 25-vitamin D postsurgery can no doubt assist in recovery, speed weight loss, and prevent this potentially devastating bone weakness and density loss.

Chronic Kidney Disease

This is not as uncommon as you might think. Chronic kidney disease affects one third of the population, about the same number of people who are obese. It's mainly seen in African Americans and is mostly due to hypertension, which, again, is a risk factor for vitamin D deficiency. The sad part about kidney disease is that it runs silently through the first three of five stages, so by the time a person is diagnosed, the prognosis can be bleak.

All patients with chronic kidney disease should be receiving vitamin D supplementation so they maintain a blood level of 25-vitamin D of at least 30 nanograms per milliliter; a blood level of up to 100 nanograms per milliliter is safe. The exact form of treatment will vary depending on the patient's baseline vitamin D status. When I treat vitamin D deficiency in patients who are on dialysis, for example, I typically administer 50,000 IU of vitamin D once a week for eight weeks as an oral capsule, and once their blood level of 25-vitamin D passes 30 nanograms per milliliter, I maintain their vitamin D status by placing them on 50,000 IU of vitamin D_2 once every two weeks. (This is what the National Kidney Foundation, in its so-called KDOQI guidelines, recommends.)

If you are diagnosed with chronic kidney disease, your doctor will likely perform a 25-vitamin D test. Have a discussion about how to safely bring your levels up, which you will certainly benefit from. For more information about chronic kidney disease as it relates to vitamin D, go to www.drholicksdsolution.com and the National Kidney Foundation's Web site (www.kidney.org). For patients with stage 3, 4, or 5 kidney disease, their kidneys may not be able to produce enough activated

vitamin D, and thus they may need to be treated with activated vitamin D (calcitriol) or one of the active vitamin D analogs that include
paracalcitriol and 1-hydroxyvitamin D_2. But even these patients need
vitamin D, as well, to keep their blood level of 25-vitamin D above 30
nanograms per milliliter.

Over-the-Counter and Prescription Drug Alerts

While there are no negative interactions with vitamin D supplements
and medications, certain medications and even some over-the-counter
herbal remedies can interfere with the body's ability to maintain robust
levels of 25-vitamin D. Here's the rundown.

Antiseizure medications. Drugs used to treat epilepsy ultimately
destroy 25-vitamin D, making patients who are on antiseizure medications
at higher risk for developing vitamin D deficiency and osteomalacia or rickets. Often two to three times as much vitamin D is required to maintain
a blood level of 25-vitamin D above 30 nanograms per milliliter; 2,000
to 6,000 IU of vitamin D a day is usually needed. An alternative, under a
doctor's care, is to take 50,000 IU of vitamin D_2 either once every week or
once every two weeks, depending on the serum 25-vitamin D level. You
want this level to be between 30 and 100 nanograms per milliliter.

Prednisone. Similarly, prednisone, an anti-inflammatory and steroid used to treat a variety of conditions, will increase the destruction of
25-vitamin D, requiring patients to increase their vitamin D intake as
well as their calcium, as prednisone also decreases calcium absorption
in the gut.

Immunotherapy. There have been a few studies looking at vitamin
D status in immunocompromised patients, including those who have had
organ transplantation (heart, lung, and kidney) and those who suffer from
AIDS. The medications that these patients are on increase the destruc-
tion of vitamin D, giving them a higher risk of vitamin D deficiency.
These patients often have significant bone loss, causing osteoporosis.
Thus, patients who are on immunotherapy or are immunocompromised
should have their vitamin D status evaluated and appropriately treated.

Often these patients need twice as much vitamin D to correct their vitamin D deficiency, and I therefore typically place them on 50,000 IU of vitamin D_2 once a week for sixteen weeks, followed by 50,000 IU of vitamin D_2 once a week or once every two weeks to maintain their blood level of 25-vitamin D above 30 nanograms per milliliter. (For more information, go to my Web site, www.drholicksdsolution.com.)

St. John's wort. This popular herbal supplement, touted as a brain booster, will enhance the destruction of 25-vitamin D in the body. If you take this herb consistently, at a minimum I would recommend being on at least 2,000 IU of vitamin D a day and having your blood level of 25-vitamin D monitored. This goes to show that the simplest things you could be taking, including seemingly harmless over-the-counter herbal remedies, can affect your ability to absorb vitamin D.

Obesity-related drugs. Patients on orlistat, a drug marketed as Xenical or Alli, are at increased risk of vitamin D deficiency because the drug decreases absorption of vitamin D (and of dietary fats—the purpose of the drug). For these patients, I recommend that they increase their vitamin D intake from 2,000 IU of vitamin D per day to 3,000 to 4,000 IU of vitamin D per day. Discuss this with your doctor if you take this medication.

Cholestyramine (brand name Questran). Used to lower cholesterol, this drug can also interfere with the absorption of vitamin D. People who take this drug over the long term to lower cholesterol should discuss with their doctor upping their vitamin D intake, and at the very least should request a 25-vitamin D test. They should take their vitamin D supplement at least two—and preferably up to four—hours after taking cholestyramine.

Et Cetera: Still Other Causes
of Vitamin D Deficiency

Some people have genetic problems or malfunctions in their kidneys or liver that prevent their bodies from making the active form of vitamin

D that benefits health. Remember, these are the key organs to the production of activated vitamin D in the body. Here are more reasons why some people may have a vitamin D deficiency that requires more aggressive treatment than the normal protocol.

Fat malabsorption syndromes. People whose ability to absorb dietary fat is compromised (fat malabsorption) may need to get their extra vitamin D from sun or tanning-bed exposure or from the FDA-sanctioned vitamin D–producing Sperti lamp. Some causes of fat malabsorption are pancreatic enzyme deficiency, Crohn's disease, cystic fibrosis, celiac disease (sprue), liver disease, surgical removal of part or all of the stomach, and small-bowel disease. Multiple surgeries for Crohn's, for example, can leave a much smaller bowel; I once had a patient whose resected bowel (reduced to just two feet) required the use of a tanning bed to get his vitamin D levels up and maintained. Symptoms of fat malabsorption include diarrhea and greasy and smelly stools. Patients with cystic fibrosis often have a difficult time absorbing vitamin D, and my colleagues and I showed that exposure to the Sperti lamp was effective in raising their blood levels of 25-vitamin D.

Crohn's disease. Patients with Crohn's disease, especially of the proximal small intestine, often have difficulty absorbing vitamin D. I take three approaches in treating and preventing vitamin D deficiency in Crohn's patients. The first approach is to give 50,000 IU of vitamin D_2 once a week or twice a week for at least eight weeks to see if the vitamin D deficiency can be corrected. Here, too, I use the trick of having the patient cut the capsule in half and place it in milk, orange juice, or some other drink and then drink the content but not the capsule. The second approach is to give much higher doses of vitamin D—starting with as much as 50,000 IU once a day until the serum 25-vitamin D reaches a level between 30 to 100 nanograms per milliliter and then tailoring the dose to maintain this blood level. The third alternative is to have the patient either go to a tanning salon or buy a vitamin D–producing lamp such as the Sperti lamp, which can be purchased at www.sperti.com. We showed that a patient with only two feet of small intestine left responded very well to being exposed three times a week to our tanning bed for 50 percent of the time recommended for tanning (wearing sun protection on her face). All of the aches and pains in her bones and muscles associated with vitamin D deficiency vanished, and her quality of life markedly improved after three months. We were able to maintain her at a normal 25-vitamin D level by exposing her to the tanning bed once or twice a week thereafter.

Kidney failure. Severe kidney disease can interfere with the conversion of 25-vitamin D to activated vitamin D. But someone with compromised kidneys would still need adequate vitamin D to benefit from all its other health benefits and support the local production of activated vitamin D in parathyroid glands to help control the parathyroid hormone levels, which usually increase in patients with stages 4 and 5 kidney disease.

Vitamin D–dependent rickets (types 1, 2, and 3). Type 1 rickets affects the body's ability to convert 25-vitamin D to its active form, 1,25-vitamin D, and type 2 interferes with the body's ability to recognize 1,25-vitamin D. Type 3 makes too much of a protein that prevents vitamin D from working. All of these patients need to take vitamin D and may also benefit from taking 1,25-vitamin D (calcitriol); this is especially true for type 1.

Seizure disorders (epilepsy). As I explained just above, long-term treatment with anticonvulsant medications, such as phenytoin and phenobarbital, can increase destruction of 25-vitamin D.

Celiac disease. It's estimated that up to 10 percent of the population has silent celiac disease (sprue). The first time many of these people notice they have a problem is when they find out they are vitamin D deficient but do not respond to therapy, especially from supplementation. Patients with celiac disease often have trouble absorbing fat-soluble vitamins, including vitamin D. And unless these patients are getting enough UVB to maintain healthy levels of vitamin D, they will become vitamin D deficient—even when taking vitamin D supplements. Vitamin D deficiency is very common in patients with celiac disease. I have found that patients with celiac disease who are appropriately treated with a gluten-free diet and who are treated for their vitamin D deficiency have significant improvement in their feeling of well-being, improvement in muscle strength, and a decrease in aches and discomfort in their bones. The initial dose of vitamin D that I recommend for my patients is 50,000 IU of vitamin D_2 once a week for eight weeks to fill the empty vitamin D tank and achieve a blood level of 25-vitamin D above 30 nanograms per milliliter. I then maintain the tank on full by giving them either 50,000 IU of vitamin D_2 once every two weeks or 2,000 IU of vitamin D_2 or vitamin D_3 daily.

Eating disorders. People with anorexia or bulimia routinely score low on bone density, can show signs of osteopenia (the prelude to the more severe osteoporosis), and may have low vitamin D levels. I advise that these patients receive 50,000 IU of vitamin D_2 once every two weeks from their doctor to maintain vitamin D sufficiency. Monitoring their blood levels of 25-vitamin D is also a must to ensure that it remains above 30 nanograms per milliliter. Obviously, putting an end to the eating disorder should also be on the agenda.

Liver failure. Liver failure decreases production of 25-vitamin D, especially when more than 80 percent of the liver is destroyed. Liver disease also makes it difficult for the intestine to absorb fat as well as vitamin D, calling for more aggressive administration of vitamin D. The associated fat malabsorption in mild to moderate liver patients is a major cause of vitamin D deficiency.

Primary biliary cirrhosis. This disease causes destruction of the bile ducts, preventing bile from reaching the intestines, where it's important for absorbing vitamin D. I treat these patients with 50,000 IU of vitamin D once or twice a week if necessary.

Cystic fibrosis. Also a disease that leads to fat malabsorption and vitamin D deficiency, cystic fibrosis calls for aggressive vitamin D_2 treatment and/or exposure to UVB radiation such as that found in a Sperti lamp. The Cystic Fibrosis Foundation's practice guidelines now call for this protocol, given studies that demonstrate its beneficial effects on improving patients' vitamin D status.

Anyone who suffers from any of the above conditions should discuss their vitamin D status with their doctor and take action to rectify the problem with high doses of vitamin D under a doctor's care.

Other causes. Patients with hyperparathyroidism and elevated serum calcium are often advised not to take any vitamin D because of worsening hypercalcemia. This, however, is incorrect. Two studies have shown that correcting vitamin D deficiency does not increase serum calcium levels but instead can help to decrease calcium and parathyroid levels. Thus, it's important to correct vitamin D deficiency in these patients.

Other causes of vitamin D deficiency due to hypersensitivity to vitamin D include patients with chronic granulomatous disorders, such as sarcoidosis, tuberculosis, and fungal infections. These patients are at an increased risk of developing vitamin D deficiency because their immune systems are activating vitamin D. They need to be treated for their vitamin D deficiency but receive much less vitamin D than patients who are otherwise normal and being treated for a deficiency; otherwise, they can suffer from high calcium in their urine and blood. I typically treat these patients with enough vitamin D to maintain their blood level of 25-vitamin D between 20 and 30 nanograms per milliliter.

CHAPTER 12

Dethroning the Cover-Up

Another giant leap for medicine and mankind

My task is only beginning. When I first started working with vitamin D, I never dreamed of what I and fellow scientists would discover over the course of three decades. My first experiments to isolate the active form of vitamin D in the body were akin to coming across a partially buried weather vane sticking out of the ground. And so I started to dig . . . and dig some more, eventually unearthing an entire castle underneath filled with treasures. In the 1980s I grew increasingly concerned about the message of abstinence from the sun and its potential for causing a vitamin D deficiency epidemic. But I never imagined that we'd see such great depths of vitamin D deficiency worldwide or that pushing back with our findings against the ever-powerful antisun campaigns would be so problematic, divisive, and contentious—very much contrary to the spirit of research and development in human medicine. For me, the evidence has always been crystal clear. Now it's just overwhelming and compelling.

Despite all the recognition that I've been honored to receive, I have to admit that some of my work and resulting advice is a source of controversy and fiery rhetoric among colleagues in the field of dermatology. In 2004 I was forced to give up my position as professor of dermatology at Boston University Medical Center, a position I had held for nearly ten years. My stalwart support of sensible sun exposure just didn't jibe with the views of the chair of the department. I still don't see eye to eye with many of my fellow members of the American Academy of Dermatology. Shame on me for challenging one of the dogmas of dermatology, but think about it: what if we had never experimented with inoculating a healthy individual with a weakened or dead form of a virus to impart immunity? What if we couldn't shift our focus from spicy foods to a common bacterium in the search to understand the cause of most stomach ulcers? What if Alexander Flemming hadn't thought twice about the plate where mold was killing the bacteria that had been growing on it over a long weekend? We might not have the vaccines and antibiotics we do today to treat an array of illnesses and diseases. I am also reminded of the story about hand washing by doctors, which was pioneered by the Hungarian-born physician Ignaz Semmelweis in the mid-nineteenth century. While working at an obstetrics clinic in Vienna, Dr. Semmelweis noticed that fatal childbed (or "puerperal") fever occurred significantly more frequently in women who were assisted by medical students than in those were assisted by midwives. After realizing the students often assisted in childbirth after performing autopsies on people who had died from infections—and not washing their hands between procedures—he instigated a strict hand washing policy. But it didn't catch on right away. It took decades for Semmelweis's "theory" to earn widespread acceptance. Following an alleged nervous breakdown, Semmelweis landed in an asylum, where he died at the age of forty-seven. Years after his death, Louis Pasteur confirmed the germ theory and hand washing became the norm among doctors.

The point of all this? Perceptions mean everything. And the dermatology community has had a long time to inoculate us with *mis*perceptions.

The last time I promoted a book for the lay public, *The UV Advantage*, I found myself frequently on the defensive, perpetually shoved in the "guilty" corner without a fair trial. But it was only a matter of time. I knew the proof would eventually stack up like a pile of neglected mail to be opened and paid attention to. And unless that proof is wholeheartedly acknowledged, the consequences of avoiding it only continue to stack up . . . just like those ignored bills and dismissed correspondence.

The sun has been a vital partner in our health, but it's been demonized unfairly (and to our detriment) in the last forty years, especially since the 1970s, when the dermatology community gained momentum. Ironically, there's been a parallel relationship between the rise of the unrelenting message of this community (and the enormously profitable sunscreen industry) that you should never be exposed to direct sunlight because it's going to cause serious skin cancer and death and the rise in vitamin D deficiency. Sadly, as a result, we now have a population largely vitamin D deficient and ludicrously fearful of the sun. May this book help change that.

The good news is that after almost twenty-five years of my trying to alert the world to the vitamin D deficiency problem, people—and physicians who once pooh-poohed my advice—are finally starting to get the message. The vitamin D deficiency and insufficiency that afflict at least half of the world's population, and remain one of the most undiagnosed medical conditions, are real—and very serious. They have grave health consequences for unborn children and adults alike. And they could lie at the root of our most enigmatic and vexing health challenges. Last year, when a panel of vitamin D researchers, including Dr. Grant, the Garland brothers, and Dr. Gorham—all of whom have been mentioned in this book—published a paper that attempted to put a price tag on vitamin D deficiency in Western Europe, they concluded that raising the population's 25-vitamin D levels to 40 nanograms per milliliter could results in a savings of 187,000 million euros a year. That translates to more than $260 billion.

That's a lot of health savings, and I'd expect the numbers to be similar in America, where health-care costs continue to climb commensurate with the population's increasing need for care. Dr. Grant projected that, if mean serum 25-vitamin D levels were raised in the general population to 45 nanograms per milliliter by solar UVB radiation, the rate of premature deaths in the United States could be reduced by about four hundred thousand per year. That would translate to a significant savings in health-care costs. Dr. Grant also recently led a study to estimate the economic burden and premature death rate in Canada attributable to low 25-vitamin D. (Canadians have mean serum 25-vitamin D levels averaging only 27 nanograms per milliliter.) The study concluded that if

Canadians could increase their 25-vitamin D to 40 nanograms per milliliter, the death rate could fall by 40,600 a year, or 18 percent, and the economic burden could drop by $18.3 billion a year, or 8.7 percent.

Long considered calcium's comrade in supporting strong bones and teeth, vitamin D has been radically redefined in history and the medical books, and will continue to earn new credit that places it in its own unique category and far from every other "vitamin." In the first six months of 2009 alone—just before this book went to press—more than 2,270 studies were published referencing this vitamin of health. No doubt by the time you read this, that number will have soared to greater heights. Twenty years ago, only a small handful of studies had ever been published on the subject, and when I wrote my first book, we were standing on the verge of this incredible explosion in the research.

"Great leaps" are often talked about in scientific circles, referring to the giant leaps that propel an industry to a new paradigm—as well as launch society forward. The discovery of antibiotics, for example, could be considered a great leap in medicine. The steam engine and the invention of the lightbulb led to other kinds of leaps. Leaps can also be made within the human gene pool, such as when we broke away from our ape ancestors and learned to walk upright, and later when we constructed complex languages to communicate with far more sophistication, meaning, and precision. I believe our newfound appreciation for vitamin D constitutes a great leap forward in medicine, and I applaud the numerous investigators worldwide who today are robustly investigating this area. But to the dismay of the dermatology community, a leap we haven't experienced yet is one in our bodies' ability to thrive without a little help from the sun. We just haven't yet evolved to a point where we can make ample supplies of vitamin D without UVB. Take away access to those supplements and you'd be hard-pressed to survive.

For some, even physicians, it's incomprehensible that vitamin D can reduce the risk of heart attack by as much as 50 percent; reduce the risk of common cancers of the colon, prostate, and breast by as much as 50 percent; reduce the risk of infections diseases, including influenza, by as much as 90 percent; reduce the risk of type 1 diabetes by 78 percent in a child who gets 2,000 IU of vitamin D a day in the first year of life;

decrease the risk of type 2 diabetes; decrease the risk of dementia and depression; wipe out cases of fibromyalgia that have been misdiagnosed; and dramatically decrease the risk of multiple sclerosis and other auto-immune diseases. When in doubt, I always go back to this simple fact: every tissue and cell in the body has a vitamin D receptor. Why would they be there if they weren't having an effect? We are gradually coming to an understanding that perhaps all cells in our bodies respond posi-tively to activated vitamin D, raising the prospect of an untold number of benefit associated with exposure to UVB radiation from natural or artificial sources.

I am not suggesting that vitamin D is a cure-all, but I think that we can no longer keep our blinders on to the special bond our bodies have had with the sun in ensuring our health for millennia. The dermatol-ogy community might continue to play with its eyes half open to all the research, but now that you have the knowledge, you get to decide how to live your life. I expect lots of criticism from my fellow dermatologists, and that's fine. I'm prepared. Always have been. Those who have a vested interest in promoting sunphobia don't much care that peer-reviewed studies are being published with increasing frequency that contradict their claims. Their attitude is that most people don't read these studies and any news of them in the mainstream media can be quashed with another "Stay out of the sun!" and "Cover up!" campaign accompanied by vague recommendations to just eat and drink more fortified foods and milk (which, of course, can't provide nearly enough vitamin D to benefit health). Think about it: our bodies evolved during a time when we spent most of our days outside, making in our skin an amount of vitamin D equivalent to ingesting 10,000 to 20,000 IU a day. Today, as most of us hunker down indoors, we get maybe a measly few hundred IU from diet sources. That cannot even make a dent in filling our empty tanks—a trickle in a well run dry. Don't be fooled by geography. Recall that 87 percent of dermatologists in a place as sunny as Australia—the skin cancer capital of the world—have been shown to be deficient in the summer, prompting the Australian College of Dermatologists, Austra-lian and New Zealand Bone and Mineral Society, Osteoporosis Austra-lia, and the Cancer Council Australia to publish public health alerts and offer clear directions on how to use sensible sun exposure for optimal health.

It will be hard for anyone to dismiss the claims and research contained in this book as "unscientific." They all arise from peer-reviewed studies published in prestigious medical journals. This means that when they were submitted for publication, the studies were scrutinized by a relentless and conscientious panel of doctors and scientists who carefully judged them based on how sound their methodology was, the importance of their results to the particular area of science, and how well they were executed. Only a very small percentage of studies submitted to medical journals are accepted for publication. The fact so many have been published on vitamin D in the last five years alone says something significant. Extremely significant.

Which brings me to why I've included such an extensive bibliography (coming up at the back of this book). I want you to have all the facts at your disposal. You can read more about these studies by searching the names of the papers on the National Library of Medicine's Web site (key word: pubmed) or simply going to www.pubmed.com. As more studies are published, I will be featuring them on my Web site, www.drholicksdsolution.com, so please feel free to visit and see what's new in this exciting field.

I believe Charles Schulz said it the best in his *Peanuts* comic strip, in the cartoon where Linus is sitting in the school yard and opens his lunch to find a note from his mother in which she encourages him to "make good friends, get good grades" and notes, "I hope that you are sitting in the sun, for a little sun is good as long as we don't over do it. Perhaps 10 minutes a day this time of the year is about right." Schulz was right on target for someone living in San Diego. Hopefully this message will be heard and this recommendation will be adopted worldwide.

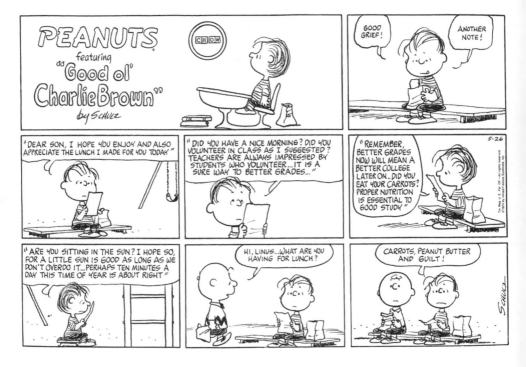

Figure 8. This witty *Classic Peanuts* comic strip first appeared in 1974, and remains as relevant as ever. Charles Schultz lived in San Diego and the recommendation that Linus receives from his mother to sit in the sun for a few minutes at that latitude is right on target. (Peanuts: United Feature Syndicate, Inc.)

CHAPTER 13

Q & A

Odds and ends and a few more reminders
in the classic FAQ style

Following are answers to some frequently asked questions I get from the lay and academic communities alike. In many of these answers you'll find echoes of information from previous sections of the book, and at times I will refer back to those pages. If you have a question not answered below, just log on to my Web site, www.drholicksdsolution .com and ask me there. You'll find other Q & As on the site, too.

General

Q. What happens when you cook foods rich in Vitamin D, like wild salmon? Do they lose their potency?
   A. Vitamin D is relatively stable in foods. Storage, processing, and cooking have little effect on its activity. Vitamin D is stable when heated to boiling temperature of 212°F.

Q. If you fry fish in oil, does that remove the vitamin D?
   A. Yes, more than 50 percent of the vitamin D is lost when you fry fish in oil. You would do well to bake, broil, or grill the fish.

Q. Does vitamin D interact with any medications?
   A. Vitamin D does not interact with any medications. However, some medications, such as antiseizure drugs, AIDS medications,

and prednisone, will increase the destruction of 25-vitamin D, thus requiring patients to increase their vitamin D intake (see chapter 11).

Q. Does genetics play a role in the ability to maintain 25-vitamin D levels?

A. There is some evidence that genetics does play a small role in the ability to maintain vitamin D status. However, from my experience, if you ingest between 1,500 and 2,000 IU of vitamin D a day, and you are not obese, this often will satisfy your vitamin D requirement.

Q. Can you receive vitamin D from sunlight through windows? What impact does cloud cover have?

A. Sunlight coming through window glass will not produce any vitamin D in the skin because the glass absorbs the vitamin D–producing UVB radiation. Your skin must be exposed to direct sunlight in order to make vitamin D. Cloud cover will decrease the amount of UVB radiation penetrating to the earth and can reduce vitamin D_3 synthesis by as much as 50 percent to 75 percent.

Q. Is there an age at which vitamin D supplementation doesn't work?

A. Absolutely not. Vitamin D supplementation is effective in children and adults of all ages. Aging does not affect the body's ability to absorb vitamin D either from the diet or from supplements. At least 1,000 IU of vitamin D day is appropriate for all ages, from children one year old to geriatric patients. Newborns during the first year of life should take at least 400 IU a day, and up to 1,000 IU is reasonable.

Q. Does aging affect my ability to make vitamin D in my skin?

A. Yes, but the skin has such a large capacity that even with a 70 percent reduction by the time you're seventy years old, you can still make enough just by exposing more skin.

Q. I have heard that it is important to take magnesium along with vitamin D. Is there any reason for this?

A. There is no need to take magnesium along with vitamin D. Vitamin D is efficiently absorbed with or without magnesium.

Q. How much calcium should you have with 1,000 IU of vitamin D a day?

A. The Institute of Medicine recommends that all adults up to the age of fifty ingest 1,000 milligrams of calcium a day and adults over the age of fifty 1,200 milligrams of calcium a day. Teenagers require 1,300 milligrams a day to maximize their bone health.

Q. Is it okay to take vitamin D without taking calcium supplements?

A. Yes. However, to maximize vitamin D's effect on skeletal health, you need to ingest, either from supplements or from diet, 1,000 to 1,200 milligrams of calcium a day depending on your age (see chapter 9). Teens need even more—1,300 milligrams a day.

Q. Do carbonated beverages affect vitamin D or calcium levels?

A. No. Carbonated beverages do not affect vitamin D or calcium levels.

Q. Should you stop taking vitamin D supplements just before having your vitamin D status checked?

A. There is no need to stop your vitamin D to have your 25-vitamin D level checked.

Q. How do you interpret different vitamin D lab numbers (i.e., do you look at 25-vitamin D_2, 25-vitamin D_3, or total 25-vitamin D)?

A. When you check the blood level of 25-vitamin D, the only number that is important is the total 25-vitamin D, which should be above 30 nanograms per milliliter. The 25-vitamin D_2 level reflects vitamin D_2 intake (usually from a vitamin D_2 prescription), and the

25-vitamin D_3 level reflects the vitamin D_3 ingested from diet, supplements, and sun exposure. Adding together the 25-vitamin D_2 and 25-vitamin D_3 numbers gives the total 25-vitamin D number. For example, if your results show a vitamin D_2 number of 15 nanograms per milliliter and a vitamin D_3 count of 20 nanograms per milliliter, then your total vitamin D would be 35 nanograms per milliliter.

Q. Is it possible to get vitamin D toxicity with vitamin D supplementation and a diet high in vitamin D–fortified foods along with sun exposure?

A. In my opinion, because very few foods contain vitamin D and the amount of vitamin D is relatively small in comparison to what the body requires, it is doubtful that you could become vitamin D toxic by taking a vitamin D supplement of 1,000 to 2,000 IU of vitamin D a day. You cannot get too much from the sun, either. Most of the literature suggests that adults have to ingest more than 10,000 IU of vitamin D a day for at least five months before they have to begin to be concerned about vitamin D toxicity. If you have sarcoidosis or another granulomatous disorder like tuberculosis, you could be more sensitive to vitamin D and need to check with your doctor.

Q. Is farmed salmon a good source of vitamin D?

A. My colleagues and I found that farmed salmon has only about 10 percent to 25 percent of the vitamin D found in wild-caught salmon. We have tested the Vital Choice wild-caught salmon available at www.vitalchoice.com and found that it has between 800 and 1,000 IU of vitamin D in 3.5 ounces.

Q. Why do some textbooks still call vitamin D the most toxic vitamin?

A. Indeed, most textbooks still call vitamin D the most toxic vitamin. It definitely is not. Vitamin A is much more toxic and can rapidly cause death in very high concentrations. (This was discovered by early explorers in Alaska who began eating polar bear liver and became severely vitamin A intoxicated, leading to death.) Given the plethora of data emerging on the safety of vitamin D, I expect the textbooks may be rewritten.

Q. Should children who do not drink much milk and who wear sunscreen get their blood levels of 25-vitamin D checked?

A. It's not unreasonable to have your children tested if you are concerned about their being vitamin D deficient because they don't drink milk or wear sunscreen all the time. This will help convince you and the pediatrician that the child is vitamin D deficient and requires vitamin D treatment. However, because this test is rather costly, I often recommend that children simply take 1,000 IU of vitamin D a day along with a multivitamin containing 400 IU of vitamin D a day.

Q. Does time of day matter for recommended sun exposure?

A. The time of day does matter, because the angle of the sun is different. It's very difficult to make vitamin D in the early morning or late afternoon, even in the summer, and you will make more vitamin D between noon and 2:00 P.M. than you will either make at 10:00 A.M. or 3:00 P.M. (see tables starting on page 182).

Q. Are there any vitamin D–stimulating lightbulbs for humans?

A. Vitamin D will not be produced by exposure to incandescent lightbulbs. You need to be exposed to a vitamin D–producing lamp that emits UVB radiation. The Sperti lamp is the only FDA-sanctioned vitamin D–producing lamp. Tanning beds that have fluorescent lamps also emit UVB radiation.

Q. Does it matter whether I wear sunglasses when I expose myself to the sun?

A. I always recommend some face protection and sunglasses or other eye protection to reduce the risk of cataracts.

Q. Does boiling cow's milk destroy vitamin D?

A. Boiling cow's milk will not destroy vitamin D. Vitamin D is heat stable at least up to a temperature of about 300°F.

Q. Is vitamin D better absorbed from fortified dairy or from fortified juice?

A. My colleagues and I have recently completed a study with Minute Maid fortified orange juice finding that vitamin D is equally bioavailable from fortified juice, fortified milk, and vitamin D supplement capsules.

Q. I've heard that vitamin D in skim or nonfat milk isn't as bioavailable. Is this true?

A. Vitamin D is just as bioavailable from skim and nonfat milk as it is from whole milk. Fat is not needed to efficiently absorb vitamin D.

Q. Isn't vitamin D fat soluble? Is there a water-soluble form of vitamin D that is used to fortify orange juice and skim milk?

A. The vitamin D that is used in orange juice is in a micronized form that makes it water soluble. The vitamin D in skim milk is the same vitamin D that is in whole milk and is perfectly bioavailable.

Q. Will I wash off the vitamin D I produce in my skin if I take a bath or shower within thirty minutes of being exposed to sunlight?

A. No. Vitamin D is made in living cells in the skin. You cannot wash it off!

Dosage

Q. How long does it take to increase 25-vitamin D levels after starting supplementation?

A. From my experience, healthy adults taking 1,000 IU of vitamin D a day reach their peak blood level within five to six weeks. When I treat patients with 50,000 IU of vitamin D_2 once a week for eight weeks to treat a deficiency, their blood level begins to increase by the first week and levels off by the eighth week of treatment.

Q. Is there any advantage to taking smaller doses more frequently rather than one large dose per day?

A. There is no advantage to taking smaller doses more frequently rather than a large dose of 1,000 or 2,000 IU of vitamin D a day. Indeed, you can take 2,000 IU of vitamin D a day or 14,000 IU of vitamin D once a week or 60,000 IU of vitamin D once a month; they all work the same way. I like to give my patients 50,000 IU of vitamin D_2 once every two weeks, but if they forget, taking 100,000 IU once a month is safe.

Q. Do you need to take a supplement even during the summer?

A. If you're good about getting plenty of sensible sun exposure throughout the summer months, or you live in a sunny place like Florida, then you may not necessarily need to supplement. However, it's much easier to get into the routine of taking a supplement year-round. And even Floridians have been shown to be largely deficient, because they avoid the sun or wear sun protection. You cannot overdose on sunlight exposure and become vitamin D intoxicated, so no matter how much sun you get during the summer, taking an additional 1,000 to 2,000 IU supplement cannot hurt you. I recommend that everyone take 1,000 to 2,000 IU of vitamin D a day along with a multivitamin containing 400 IU of vitamin D. This will not cause any buildup of vitamin D in the body, and by using this routine, you are less likely to forget it in the winter. I personally take 2,000 IU a day plus a multivitamin and three glasses of milk. If you are obese or have fat malabsorption syndrome due to an underlying medical condition, you may need two to three times as much (see chapter 10).

Q. How many units of vitamin D would a person have to take to become toxic?

A. Vitamin D intoxication will not occur until a person is taking more than 10,000 IU of vitamin D a day for more than six months. Adults who received 10,000 IU of vitamin D a day for five months showed no signs of toxicity. You cannot over-dose on vitamin D from exposure to sunlight or a tanning bed or a UVB-producing lamp, no matter how much UVB you get.

Q. What is the best supplement for children who cannot swallow pills?

A. Infants can be administered vitamin D through pediatric vita-min drops (see the Resource Guide). If you have children who cannot or will not swallow pills, you can crush a vitamin D tablet or squeeze the contents of a gel capsule into a glass of milk or juice. A good product that has emerged on the market and that I have used for my young patients is a liquid form of vitamin D. Made by Wellesse, it contains 500 IU of vitamin D per tea-spoon.

Q. Does the recommended dose of vitamin D supplement need to be taken with fat (not in a tablet form)?

A. The recommended dose of vitamin D supplement does not need to be taken with fat. My lab has shown that vitamin D is equally bioavailable in corn oil, milk, and orange juice.

Q. How should a vegan or vegetarian make sure he or she gets enough vitamin D?

A. Vegans should supplements with at least 1,000 IU of vitamin D a day, and preferably 2,000 IU. This would be in addition to a multivitamin. Vegans concerned about animal sources of supple-mental vitamin D_3 can opt for supplements containing vitamin D_2, which comes from yeast.

Q. What is your advice for vegan or vegetarian children?

A. I recommend that all children, including vegan children, ingest at least 400 IU of vitamin D a day, and preferably 1,000 IU of vitamin D a day, along with a multivitamin, especially if they are not getting adequate exposure to sunlight.

Q. If a person is not vitamin D deficient, what is the best over-the-counter form and dose to take? What if the person *is* vitamin D deficient?

A. If a person is not vitamin D deficient, to maintain vitamin D sufficiency I recommend that the person take at least 1,000 IU of vitamin D_2 or 1,000 IU of vitamin D_3 a day in addition to a multivitamin with 400 IU of vitamin D. If a person is vitamin D deficient, then I double or triple the dose and recommend that he or she take 2,000 to 3,000 IU of vitamin D a day along with a multivitamin. A person who is severely vitamin D deficient should consult a doctor to inquire about prescription-level treatment (see chapter 10 for more details).

Q. What form of supplementation do you recommend—D_2 or D_3?

A. In my experience, 1,000 IU of vitamin D_2 is as effective as 1,000 IU of vitamin D_3 in raising blood levels of 25-vitamin D. Either form can be used. But note: to raise blood levels of 25-vitamin D to above 30 nanograms per milliliter, you need to take more than 1,000 IU.

Q. Is the prescription form of vitamin D different from what's available over the counter?

A. In the United States, the only vitamin D form available by prescription is vitamin D_2, also known as ergocalciferol. It comes either in a capsule with 50,000 IU of vitamin D_2 or in a liquid form (for pediatric patients) with 8,000 IU of vitamin D_2 per 1 milliliter. Vitamin D_2 can also be found in some over-the-counter supplements, and it's just as effective as D_3.

Q. What is the best supplement brand?

A. Any national brand will do. For a list of ideas, see the Resource Guide.

Q. Can a prescription dose of 50,000 IU of vitamin D_2 (to correct deficiency) cause fatigue?

A. I do find that some of my patients who take 50,000 IU of vitamin D$_2$ feel fatigued. I believe that this may be due to the gelatin capsule rather than to the 50,000 IU of vitamin D$_2$. Try cutting the capsule, dumping it into milk or orange juice, and drinking the content without the capsule.

Q. Are there side effects from taking 50,000 IU at one time?

A. In my experience, there are no side effects from taking 50,000 IU of vitamin D$_2$ at one time. However, some patients are not able to tolerate it or have some GI issues. I believe that this is due to the gelatin capsule, not the vitamin D. For these patients, I recommend that they cut the capsule open, dump it into a glass of milk or orange juice, and drink the contents without the capsule.

Q. What does vitamin D toxicity look like?

A. Vitamin D toxicity is often difficult to diagnose. The diagnosis is made based on the blood biochemistries that include elevated blood calcium (usually above 10.4 milligrams per deciliter) along with a markedly elevated level of 25-vitamin D, usually above 200 nanograms per milliliter. The hypercalcemia and often hyperphosphatemia associated with vitamin D intoxication can cause the kidneys to calcify, increase the risk of developing kidney stones, and increase the risk of calcifying blood vessels (which ultimately can lead to death). The elevated blood calcium also causes constipation, confusion, depression, increased thirst, increased urination, and changes in the electrocardiogram.

Q. What is the safest way for toddlers to ingest vitamin D pills? Should an infant's or toddler's blood level of 25-vitamin D be the same as an adult's?

A. For infants and toddlers, Poly Vi-Sol is a liquid vitamin supplement that contains 400 IU of vitamin D per milliliter. Alternatively, I have suggested to parents that they can buy the 1,000 IU vitamin D tablet, grind it up, put it into the toddler's orange juice or milk, and then have him or her drink it. Or you can purchase the liquid form of vitamin D from Wellesse (available at Costco's drugstore or online at www.wellesse.com) and add two teaspoons (for a total of 1,000 IU) to the child's beverage of choice. All children and adults should maintain a blood level of 25-vitamin D of at least 30 nanograms per milliliter all the time. See Resource Guide for more.

Q. At what age do you recommend children start taking 1,000 IU a day? How much vitamin D do you recommend for infants?

A. I believe that all children over the age of one year should be on 1,000 IU of vitamin D a day plus a multivitamin. Infants should be on at least 400 IU of vitamin D a day, and, as I have pointed out, 1,000 IU of vitamin D a day should not cause any harm and may provide additional benefits.

Q. Do very lean people require a lower-dose supplement?

A. Normal weight people and very lean people do not require a lower dose of vitamin D. However, anorexic patients have been found to have marginally higher blood levels of 25-vitamin D from taking the same amount of vitamin D that a normal weight person would take. However, this is of little clinical significance.

Q. Do you recommend higher amounts of vitamin D supplementation for those who are obese?

A. I do recommend that obese people double or triple their intake of vitamin D, so instead of taking 1,000 to 2,000 IU of vitamin D a day they should take between 4,000 and 6,000 IU of vitamin D a day.

Q. I take fish oil capsules every day. Don't those contain vitamin D?

A. No. Fish oil capsules do not contain any vitamin D. Sold mostly for their omega-3 fatty acids, fish oil capsules are not necessarily made from vitamin D–rich fish like cod or salmon. The refining process isolates the omega-3 fatty acids, and any vitamin D present is left behind, which is why you don't see any vitamin D (or vitamin A, for that matter) listed on the label.

Q. I don't mind cod liver oil. Why can't I just rely on that?

A. Because of the high vitamin A content of cod liver oil, it's not a good idea to down lots of it and risk vitamin A toxicity. If you enjoy cod liver oil, stick to a single serving and seek additional vitamin D through sensible sun exposure or supplements.

Pregnancy and Newborns

Q. What are your recommendations for vitamin D during pregnancy?

A. I recommend that all pregnant women take a prenatal vitamin that contains 400 IU of vitamin D a day along with a vitamin D supplement of 1,000 IU a day. Their calcium supplements may also contain 400 IU of vitamin D. At a minimum, all pregnant women should be taking at least 1,400 IU of vitamin D a day, and 2,000 IU of vitamin D day is fine, especially for obese women. They should have a blood level of 25-vitamin D between 30 and 100 nanograms per milliliter.

Q. What is your recommendation for dispensing vitamin D to breastfeeding infants?

A. The American Academy of Pediatrics recently came out with the recommendation that all infants, including breastfed infants, should receive 400 IU of vitamin D a day. Although I agree with this recommendation, this is the bare minimum. Remember, 2,000 IU a day during the first year of life can decrease a child's risk of diabetes by nearly 80 percent. Thus, giving infants 1,000 IU a day may be more beneficial to their health.

Q. If a woman is already taking 400 IU of vitamin D in a prenatal vitamin, how much more is needed during pregnancy and breastfeeding?

A. I encourage all pregnant and lactating women to take the prenatal vitamin containing 400 IU of vitamin D a day along with
an additional 1,000 IU vitamin D supplement, for a total of at
least 1,400 IU of vitamin D a day. They should also take calcium
supplements (1,000 milligrams a day, which can be split into two
servings of 500 milligrams each). Or they can obtain their calcium by drinking three to four glasses of skim milk or calcium-
fortified orange juice, which will likely be fortified with vitamin
D, too. I believe that pregnant and lactating women can easily
take 2,000 IU of vitamin D a day without causing any toxicity.
They should maintain a blood level of 25-vitamin D between 30
and 100 nanograms per milliliter.

Q. **We used to think too much vitamin D in pregnant women would
cause the fetus's head growth to be stunted. Is that a myth?**
A. Yes, it is a myth. I'm not sure what you mean by "too much vitamin D," but certainly taking the recommended 1,400 to 2,000 IU
of vitamin D a day will not stunt the fetus's head growth. Vitamin
D *deficiency* in utero, however, can.

Q. **Why are infants only to receive 400 IU? How about premature infants?**
A. Infants appear to satisfy most of their vitamin D requirement for
bone health by receiving 400 IU of vitamin D a day. This is the recommendation made by the American Academy of Pediatrics and the
Canadian Pediatric Society. There is some evidence that premature
infants may not be able to metabolize vitamin D as efficiently, but
there are no data to suggest that giving a premature infant more
than 400 IU of vitamin D a day has any additional benefit. Thus, I
would recommend that infants, including premature infants, receive
at least 400 IU of vitamin D a day, and I believe that up to 1,000 IU
of vitamin D a day is safe for them.

Q. **I am in my third trimester and have been supplementing with
1,400 IU of vitamin D$_3$ a day. My doctor wants me to stop**

supplementing because my levels of activated vitamin D are twice normal and my 25-vitamin D is normal. She's worried about toxicity. Should I be?

A. Absolutely not. Activated vitamin D (1,25-vitamin D) goes up during the second and third trimester; this is in response to your body's making more vitamin D–binding protein and your need to increase your efficiency of absorbing dietary supplemental calcium for fetal mineralization. You are perfectly fine and should continue to take your vitamin D. You and your baby will benefit.

Disease, Disorders, and Special Conditions

Q. Once you are diagnosed with cancer, does it help to take vitamin D supplements?

A. We don't know whether increasing vitamin D once a diagnosis of cancer is made provides any benefit in reducing the growth of the cancer or the cancer's outcome. However, there is no reason not to have all cancer patients take enough vitamin D to maintain their blood level of 25-vitamin D between 30 and 100 nanograms per milliliter. It may improve muscle strength and bone strength as well as possibly enhancing the therapeutic benefit of any cancer treatment. Patients with cancer often have aches and pains in their bones, muscles, and joints, as well as gastrointestinal upset. Curing them of a vitamin D deficiency can help. My studies have shown that cancer patients are typically deficient. We have also demonstrated in mice that colon and prostate cancer cell growth is less in mice receiving adequate vitamin D.

Q. Are vitamin D supplements safe during chemotherapy, or could they interact with the action of these agents?

A. There is no evidence that vitamin D supplements will interact with chemotherapy. Therefore, vitamin D supplementation is safe during chemotherapy. My lab has found that more than 50 percent of patients with various cancers who were on chemotherapy were severely vitamin D sufficient.

Q. Is it necessary to have 25-vitamin D levels between 60 and 80 nanograms per milliliter to prevent cancer?
A. It does appear that a blood level of 25-vitamin D is at least 30 nanograms per milliliter may decrease the risk of many deadly cancers. It is unknown, however, the blood level needs to be 60 nanograms per milliliter. There is no harm in keeping the blood level at between 60 and 80 nanograms per milliliter. I have all of my patients on enough vitamin D to maintain their blood levels between 40 and 100 nanograms per milliliter, which I believe to be both therapeutic and preventative of chronic diseases including common cancers.

Q. Is vitamin D deficiency linked to thyroid disease?
A. Vitamin D deficiency does not cause thyroid disease, but patients with hyperthyroidism (an overactive thyroid that leads to an imbalance of the body's metabolic hormones, tripping a cascade of health problems) have increased destruction of 25-vitamin D and are at higher risk of vitamin D deficiency (see chapter 11).

Q. Is there any correlation between vitamin D deficiency and hypothyroidism (an underactive thyroid)?
A. There is no correlation between vitamin D deficiency and hypothyroidism. Vitamin D deficiency is so common that often patients with hypothyroidism are also vitamin D deficient. All patients, including hypothyroid patients, should be treated for their vitamin D deficiency and prevent vitamin D deficiency by staying on an adequate amount of vitamin D.

Q. When children raised in equatorial areas move to the United States and develop high rates of autism, could this be related to Vitamin D deficiency?
A. There is little information regarding the cause of autism, and there has been a suggestion that vitamin D deficiency may increase

risk of it. However, to date there have not been any clinical trials demonstrating that vitamin D improves autism. However, it is important that everyone, including children with autism, have an adequate amount of vitamin D to maintain their blood level of 25-vitamin D of between 30 and 100 nanograms per milliliter.

Q. Is there any evidence that treating patients with autoimmune diseases with vitamin D can lessen their symptoms?

A. There are no prospective studies that have treated patients with autoimmune diseases with high doses of vitamin D, so we do not know whether such treatment would lessen their symptoms. However, vitamin D deficiency is associated with many nonspecific symptoms, including muscle weakness, muscle aches and pains, bone aches and pains, and joint aches and pains, which can be associated with autoimmune diseases including multiple sclerosis and rheumatoid arthritis. In my experience, not only does treating patients with multiple sclerosis with vitamin D improve their overall feeling of well-being and muscle strength, but some of my patients also have had an extended honeymoon from their disease. Patients with rheumatoid arthritis who are vitamin D deficient also have improvement in muscle function and decreased aches and pains in their bones and joints when the deficiency is treated.

Q. Can vitamin D help with the symptoms of multiple sclerosis (MS)? Will vitamin D supplementation delay the progression of MS in someone who has MS?

A. I have found that my patients with multiple sclerosis are often vitamin D deficient. Since vitamin D deficiency causes muscle weakness, I have found that correcting their vitamin D deficiency significantly improves overall muscle function. A few of my patients who had their first symptoms of multiple sclerosis and then were treated with 50,000 IU of vitamin D once a week for eight weeks and every other week thereafter, have remained in their honeymoon period. Thus, if you have multiple sclerosis, there is no reason not to have your vitamin D status checked, be treated for your vitamin D deficiency, and prevent the recurrence of vitamin D deficiency.

Q. In mild to moderate cases of osteopenia (the prelude to osteoporosis), would taking adequate vitamin D and calcium be enough to prevent osteoporosis, thus eliminating need for osteoporosis medications?

A. In my experience, many men and women who present with mild or moderate osteopenia are vitamin D deficient and calcium deficient. I typically treat them for their vitamin D deficiency and then maintain them on 50,000 IU of vitamin D₂ every two weeks. In addition, for adults under the age of fifty, I place them on a total of 1,000 milligrams of calcium, either from dietary sources or from supplements, and for adults over the age of fifty, I increase this by 200 milligrams, so that they ingest approximately 1,200 to 1,500 milligrams of calcium a day from diet and supplements. I recommend that the calcium be taken in two or three divided doses, rather than all at once, because it will be more bioavailable. The vitamin D can be taken any time. I follow these patients, and often after one to two years, I reevaluate their bone mineral density. Often the patients either have a small increase in their bone mineral density or no significant change. But some can have a dramatic increase of 10 percent to 15 percent if they have osteomalacia due to vitamin D deficiency. Only when I see that the bone density is reduced by more than 5 percent within a year do I become aggressive in considering giving medication to prevent osteoporosis.

Q. Does vitamin D have any association with scoliosis in adolescent girls? Can vitamin D supplementation help correct spinal curvature?

A. I am not aware of any association between scoliosis and vitamin D deficiency in adolescent girls. However, many adolescent girls are vitamin D deficient, and to maximize their bone health, they should be receiving an adequate amount of vitamin D and calcium (see box on page 204). But vitamin D supplementation will not correct spinal curvature. Unfortunately, this is a permanent deformity. But if the vitamin D deficiency is exacerbating the spinal curvature, correcting vitamin D deficiency may help prevent further curvature from occurring. Keep in mind that vitamin D will also improve muscle strength; a study out of Lebanon showed that 2,000 IU a day to girls ten to seventeen years old did just that. Another recent study, which examined the influence of low 25-vitamin D levels on bone mass, bone turnover, and muscle strength in 301 healthy Chinese adolescent girls, also confirmed the importance of adequate vitamin D in reaching peak bone mass and muscle strength.

Q. Would your recommendations be the same for Down's syndrome and intellectual disability patients?

A. I recommend that children over one year and adults receive at least 1,400 to 2,000 IU of vitamin D a day if they are not getting adequate exposure to sunlight. This also applies to patients with Down's syndrome and with intellectual disabilities. (Again, newborns should receive at least 400 IU of vitamin D, and up to 1,000 IU a day is safe and may be more beneficial.)

Q. Do any of the studies cited demonstrate an increased incidence of kidney stones in patients taking the levels of vitamin D you suggest?

A. In my opinion, there is no increased risk of developing kidney stones in patients who are treated for vitamin D deficiency and maintain vitamin D sufficiency as I have recommended. Most of the studies that have reported an association were poorly designed or poorly controlled. I have not found any increased risk of kidney stones in my patients whom I have treated vitamin D deficiency and maintained at a normal vitamin D status. I believe that this is a myth.

Q. I have primary hyperparathyroidism and my calcium is elevated and I am vitamin D deficient. My doctor says taking

vitamin D will increase my calcium level and therefore I should avoid vitamin D. True?

A. This is not true. Two studies have proved that, if anything, your parathyroid hormone and calcium levels will be improved by correcting the vitamin D deficiency.

Q. I have sarcoidosis and my doctor says I should not take vitamin D because it could cause my calcium to elevate above normal. True?

A. It is true that excessive exposure to sunlight or taking too much vitamin D can cause the macrophages in the sarcoid tissue to make too much activated vitamin D. However, patients should not remain vitamin D deficient, because that can cause muscle weakness and symptoms of osteomalacia (aches and pains in bones and muscles). I treat my sarcoidosis patients with just enough vitamin D to maintain their 25-vitamin D level between 20 and 30 nanograms per milliliter, and I monitor their serum calcium to be certain it does not elevate above the normal range.

Q. I have kidney disease and am on dialysis. My doctor said that since my kidneys cannot make activated vitamin D from 25-vitamin D, there is no need for me to take vitamin D to maintain my blood levels of 25-vitamin D above 30 nanograms per milliliter. Is this correct?

A. No. The National Kidney Foundation and I recommend that all patients with kidney failure—even patients with no kidneys—should maintain 25-vitamin D levels of 30 to 100 nanograms per milliliter.

Q. What about people who have a vitamin D receptor (VDR) defect and need more vitamin D?

A. Patients who have a VDR defect can sometimes benefit by increasing their vitamin D intake. It depends upon the severity of the alteration in the VDR gene. Patients with the VDR gene mutation known as vitamin D–resistant rickets or vitamin D–dependent rickets type II will sometimes benefit from being treated not only with vitamin D but also with the active form of vitamin D, 1,25-vitamin D.

Q. I take medications that make me extra sensitive to the sun. What should I do?

A. If you cannot expose yourself to the sun for any amount of time, then supplementation is key. Aim to take 2,000 IU of vitamin D a day year-round. This can be in addition to any multivitamin containing vitamin D, vitamin D–fortified foods and beverages, and D-rich fish you consume.

Q. A lot of women are being given gabapentin for hot flashes instead of estrogen. Can it lower 25-vitamin D levels?

A. We do not know whether gabapentin (brand name Neurontin or Gabarone) used for treating hot flashes will lower 25-vitamin D levels. However, we do know that many drugs and even St. John's wort will enhance the destruction of vitamin D in the body. Thus, at a minimum I would recommend being on at least 2,000 IU of vitamin D a day and having your blood level of 25-vitamin D monitored.

RESOURCE GUIDE

The following list of resources is intended as a guide to help you maximize the program outlined in this book. Some of these products I have done research on or have used. It is by no means exhaustive because it's impossible to list every trusted resource available to you. Explore options in your local area, and I invite you to also go to www.drholicksdsolution.com for updated information and help in finding the best products to support your health.

Vitamin D–Producing Light

Sperti Lamp mfg. by KBD, Inc.
www.vitaminduv.com
info@vitaminduv.com
859-331-0800

Wild Seafood

Vital Choice
PO Box 4121
Bellingham, WA 98227
www.vitalchoice.com
Sales Line: 800-608-4825
Customer Service: 866-482-5887

Supplement Brands

Wellesse
www.wellesse.com
1-800-232-4005

Vital Nutrients
www.vitalnutrients.com
1-888-328-9992

Lane Labs
www.lanelabs.com
1-800-526-3005

Vital Choice
PO Box 4121
Bellingham, WA 98227
www.vitalchoice.com
Sales Line: 800-608-4825
Customer Service: 866-482-5887

Perque
*Perque's "D3 Cell Guard" is sold through doctors and health-care professionals
1-800-525-7352
www.perque.com
info@perque.com

Nature Made
www.naturemade.com
1-800-276-2878

Metagenics
www.metagenics.com

New Chapter
New Chapter Bone Health vitamin D and calcium supplement
www.newchapter.com

Pediatric Vitamin Drops

Enfamil
www.enfamil.com
1-800-BABY-123 (1-800-2229-123)
Just D Infant Vitamin Drops
www.sunlightvitamins.com

D-Friendly Sunscreen (a sunscreen that permits you to make vitamin D)

D Sun Solution Sunscreen
www.dsunsolution.com
info@dsunsolution.com

Vitamin D–Fortified Products

Brands and general products to seek out at your local grocery store (you will often find that brands advertise right on the label that their product is fortified):

Minute Maid orange juice fortified with calcium and vitamin D
Vitamin D fortified milk, yogurt, cheese, and cottage cheese
Vitamin D fortified cereals
Vitamin D–fortified breads
Mushrooms and mushrooms exposed to sunlight or simulated sunlight
Vitamin D yeast
Boda vitamin energy drink with vitamin D (check out www.urstuff .com)

Light Boxes for Seasonal Affective Disorder

The following list of suppliers' Web sites is only a sampling of the available sources:

www.sunalux.com/s_lightboxes.cfm
www.verilux.com
www.consumer.philips.com
http://sunbox.com/
www.bio-light.com

SELECTED BIBLIOGRAPHY

At the time this book went to press, new studies continued to emerge backing up the claims of researchers that maintaining healthy levels of vitamin D is fundamental to optimal health. A book that showcases every single published study on vitamin D would span thousands of pages, for it's even impossible to list all the recent studies that have emerged in just the last twenty years in this book. What follows is a bibliography that highlights some of the more prominent studies published, including the ones that are featured in the book. The bibliography is divided into sections that cover various health issues addressed throughout this volume. To access more research and find related studies, visit my Web site at www.drholicksdsolution.com and check out the National Institute of Health's online publication library at www.pubmed.com.

Autoimmune Diseases (multiple sclerosis, rheumatoid arthritis, type 1 diabetes, etc.)

Cantorna MT, Hayes CE, DeLuca HF. "1,25-Dihydroxyholecalciferol inhibits the progression of arthritis in murine models of human arthritis." *Journal of Nutrition* 1998;128:68–72.

Cantorna MT, Hayes CE, DeLuca HF. "1,25-Dihydroxyvitamin D_3 reversibly blocks the progression of relapsing encephalomyelitis, a model of multiple sclerosis." *Proceedings of the National Academy of Sciences of the United States of America* 1996;93:7861–64.

Embry AF, Snowdon LR, Vieth R. "Vitamin D and seasonal fluctuations of gadolinium-enhancing magnetic resonance imaging lesions in multiple sclerosis." *Annals of Neurology* 2000;48:271–72.

EURODIAB Substudy 2 Study Group. "Vitamin D supplement in early childhood and risk for Type I (insulin-dependent) diabetes mellitus." *Diabetologia* 1999;42:51–54.

Harris SS. "Vitamin D and type 1 diabetes." *American Journal of Clinical Nutrition* 2004;79;889–90.

Hernán MA, Olek MJ, Ascherio A. "Geographic variation of MS incidence in two prospective studies of US women." *Neurology* 1999;51:1711–18.

Hyppönen E, Läärä E, Järvelin M-R, Virtanen SM. "Intake of vitamin D and risk of type 1 diabetes: A birth-cohort study." *Lancet* 2001;358:1500–1503.

Mathieu C, Badenhoop K. "Vitamin D and type 1 diabetes mellitus: State of the art. *Trends in Endocrinology and Metabolism* 2005;16:261–66.

Merlino LA, Curtis J, Mikuls TR, Cerhan JR, Criswell LA, Saag KG. Iowa "Women's health study. Vitamin D intake is inversely associated with rheumatoid arthritis." *Arthritis and Rheumatism* 2004; 50(1):72–77.

Mohr SB, Garland CF, Gorham ED, Garland FC. "The association between ultraviolet B irradiance, vitamin D status and incidence rates of type 1 diabetes in 51 regions worldwide." *Diabetologia* 2008 Aug;51(8):1391–98.

Munger KL, Zhang SM, O'Reilly E, Hernán MA, Olek MJ, Willett WC, Ascherio A. "Vitamin D intake and incidence of multiple sclerosis." *Neurology* 2004; 62(1):60–65.

Munger KL, Levin LI, Hollis BW, Howard NS, Ascheino A. "Serum 25-hydroxyvitamin D levels and risk of multiple sclerosis." *Journal of the American Medical Association* 2006; 296:2832–38.

Ponsonby AL, Lucas RM, van der Mei IA. "UVR, vitamin D and three autoimmune diseases-multiple sclerosis, type 1 diabetes, rheumatoid arthritis." *Photochemistry and Photobiology* 2005; 81:1267–75.

VanAmerongen BM, Dijkstra CD, Lips P, and Polman CH. "Multiple sclerosis and vitamin D: An update." *European Journal of Clinical Nutrition* 2004; 58(8):1095–109.

Brain Health (Alzheimer's, dementia, depression, seasonal affective disorder, schizophrenia, etc.)

Ancoli-Israel S, Martin JL, Kripke DF, Marler M, and Klauber MR. "Effect of light treatment on sleep and circadian rhythms in demented nursing home patients." *Journal of the American Geriatrics Society* 2002;50(2): 282–89.

Brainard GC, Hanifin JP, Rollag MD, Greeson, J, et al. "Human melatonin regulation is not mediated by the three cone photopic visual system." *Journal of Clinical Endocrinology and Metabolism* 2001;86(1):433–36.

Colenda CC, et al. "Phototherapy for patients with Alzheimer disease with disturbed sleep patterns: Results of a community-based pilot study." *Alzheimer Disease and Associated Disorders* 1997;11(3):175–78.

Czeisler CA, et al. "Use of bright light to treat maladaptation to night shift work and circadian rhythm sleep disorders." *Journal of Sleep Research* 1995;4(S2):70–73.

Davies G, Welham J, Chant D, Torrey EF, McGrath J. "A systematic review and meta-analysis of Northern Hemisphere season of birth studies in schizophrenia." *Schizophrenia Bulletin* 2003;29(3):587–93.

Eastman CI, et al. "Bright light treatment of winter depression." *Archives of General Psychiatry* 1998;55:883–89.

Eyles DW, Smith S, Kinobo R, Howison M, McGrath JJ. "Distribution of the Vitamin D receptor and 1α-hydroxylase in human brain." *Journal of Chemical Neuroanatomy* 2005;29:21–30.

Gloth FM, Alam W, and Hollis B. "Vitamin D vs broad spectrum phototherapy in the treatment of seasonal affective disorder." *Journal of Nutrition, Health and Aging* 1999;3:5–7.

Kendell RE, Adams W. "Exposure to sunlight, vitamin D and schizophrenia." *Schizophrenia Research* 2002;54(3):193–98.

Kripke DF. "Light treatment for nonseasonal depression: Speed, efficacy, and combined treatment. *Journal of Affective Disorders* 1998;49(2):109–17.

Lam RW, Levitt AJ (eds.). "Canadian consensus guidelines for the treatment of seasonal affective disorder: A summary of the report of the Canadian consensus group on SAD." *Canadian Journal of Diagnosis* 2000.

Levins PC, Carr DB, Fisher JE, Momtaz K, Parrish JA. "Plasma [beta]-endorphin and [beta]-lipotropin response to ultraviolet radiation." *Lancet* 1983;2(8342):166.

Lewy AJ, et al. "Morning vs. evening light treatment of patients with winter depression." *Archives of General Psychiatry* 1998;55:890–96.

McGrath J, Eyles D, Mowry B, Yolken R, Buka S. "Low maternal vitamin D as a risk factor for schizophrenia: A pilot study using banked sera." *Schizophrenia Research* 2003;63:73–78.

Mishima K, et al. "Morning bright light therapy for sleep and behavior disorders in elderly patients with dementia." *Acta Psychiatrica Scandinavica* 1994;89(1): 1–7.

Rosenthal NE. "Diagnosis and treatment of seasonal affective disorder." *Journal of the American Medical Association* 1993;270(22):2717–20.

Sato Y, Iwamoto J, Kanoko T, Satoh K. "Amelioration of osteoporosis and hypovitaminosis D by sunlight exposure in hospitalized, elderly women with

Alzheimer's Disease: A randomized controlled trial." *Journal of Bone and Mineral Research* 2005; 20:1327–33.

Terman M, Lewy AJ, Dijk DJ, Boulos Z, et al. "Light treatment for sleep disorders: Consensus report. IV. Sleep phase and duration disturbances." *Journal of Biological Rhythms* 1995;10:135–47.

Zanello SB, Jackson D, Holick MF. "Expression of the circadian clock genes clock and period 1 in human skin." *Journal of Investigative Dermatology* 2000;115(4):757–60.

Cancer (of the internal organs, e.g., breast, colon, prostate, ovarian, pancreatic, etc.)

Ahonen MH, Tenkanen L, Teppo L, Hakama M, Tuohimaa P. "Prostate cancer risk and prediagnostic serum 25-hydroxyvitamin D levels (Finland)." *Cancer Causes Control* 2000;11:847–52.

Apperly FL. "The relation of solar radiation to cancer mortality in North America." *Cancer Research* 1941;1:191–95.

Bertone-Johnson ER, Chen WY, Holick MF, et al. "Plasma 25-hydroxyvitamin D and 1,25-Dihydroxyvitamin D and risk of breast cancer." *Cancer Epidemiology, Biomarkers and Prevention* 2005;14:1991–97.

Bischoff-Ferrari HA, Giovannucci E, Willett WC, Dietrich T, Dawson-Hughes B. "Estimation of optimal serum concentrations of 25-hydroxyvitamin D for multiple health outcomes." *American Journal of Clinical Nutrition* 2006; 84:18–28.

Bodiwala D, Luscombe CJ, Liu S, Saxby M, French M, Jones PW. "Prostate cancer risk and exposure to ultraviolet radiation: Further support for the protective effect of sunlight." *Cancer Letters* 2003;192(2):145–49.

Chen TC, Holick MF. "Vitamin D and prostate cancer prevention and treatment." *Trends in Endocrinology and Metabolism* 2003;14:423–30.

Cross HS, Kallay E, Lechner D, Gerdenitsch W, et al. "Phytoestrogens and vitamin D metabolism: A new concept for the prevention and therapy of colorectal, prostate and mammary carcinoma." *Journal of Nutrition* 2004 May;134(5):1207S-1212S.

Feldman D, Zhao XY, Krishnan AV. Editorial/Mini-review: "Vitamin D and prostate cancer." *Endocrinology* 2000;141:5–9.

Feskanich JM, Fuchs CS, Kirkner GJ, Hankinson SE, et al. "Plasma vitamin D metabolites and risk of colorectal cancer in women." *Cancer Epidemiology, Biomarkers and Prevention* 2004;13(9):1502–8.

Freedman DM, Dosemeci M, McGlynn K. "Sunlight and mortality from breast, ovarian, colon, prostate, and non-melanoma skin cancer: A composite death certificate based case-control study." *Occupational and Environmental Medicine* 2002;59:257–62.

Garland CF, Garland FC, Shaw EK, Comstock GW, et al. "Serum 25-hydroxyvitamin D and colon cancer: Eight-year prospective study." *Lancet* 1989;18:1176–78.

Garland FC, Garland CF, Gorham ED, Young JF. "Geographic variation in breast cancer mortality in the United States: A hypothesis involving exposure to solar radiation." *Preventive Medicine* 1990;19:614–22.

Garland CF, Garland FC, Gorham ED, et al. "The role of vitamin D in cancer prevention." *American Journal of Public Health* 2006;96(2):252–61.

Garland CF, Gorham ED, Mohr SB, Garland FC. "Vitamin D for cancer prevention: Global perspective." *Annals of Epidemiology* 2009 Jul;19(7):468–83.

Garland CF, Gorham ED, Mohr SB, Grant WB, et al. "Vitamin D and prevention of breast cancer: Pooled analysis." *Journal of Steroid Biochemistry and Molecular Biology* 2006; 103(3–5):708–11.

Giovannucci E, Liu Y, Rimm EB, Hollis BW, et al. "Prospective study of predictors of vitamin D status and cancer incidence and mortality in men." *Journal of the National Cancer Institute* 2006;98(7):451–59.

Giovannucci E, Liu Y, Willett WC. "Cancer incidence and mortality and vitamin D in black ad white male health professionals." *Cancer Epidemiology, Biomarkers and Prevention* 2006;15(12):2467–72.

Gorham ED, Garland CF, Garland FC, et al. "Optimal vitamin D status for colorectal cancer prevention: A quantitative meta analysis." *American Journal of Preventive Medicine* 2007; 32(3):210–16.

Grant WB. "An estimate of premature cancer mortality in the U.S. due to inadequate doses of solar ultraviolet-B radiation." *Cancer* 2002;70:2861–69.

Grant WB. "How strong is the evidence that solar ultraviolet B and vitamin D reduce the risk of cancer?" *Dermato-Endocrinology* 2009;1:17–24.

Grant WB. "Lower vitamin-D production from solar ultraviolet-B irradiance may explain some differences in cancer survival rates." *Journal of the National Medical Association* 2006; 98(3):357–64.

Hanchette CL, Schwartz GG. "Geographic patterns of prostate cancer mortality." *Cancer* 1992;70:2861–69.

Holick MF. "Calcium plus vitamin D and the risk of colorectal cancer." *New England Journal of Medicine* 2006;354(21):2287.

Holick MF. "Vitamin D and sunlight: Strategies for cancer prevention and other health benefits." *Clinical Journal of the American Society of Nephrology* 2008 Sep;3(5):1548–55.

John EM, Schwartz GG, Dreon DM, Koo J. "Vitamin D and breast cancer risk: The NHANES I epidemiologic follow-up study, 1971–1975 to 1992." National Health and Nutrition Examination Survey. *Cancer Epidemiology, Biomarkers and Prevention* 1999;8:399–406.

Knight JA, Lesosky M, Barnett H, Raboud JM, Vieth R. "Vitamin D and reduced risk of breast cancer: A population-based case-control study." *Cancer Epidemiology, Biomarkers and Prevention* 2007;16(3):422–99.

Lappe JM, Travers-Gustafson D, Davies KM, Recker RR, Heaney RP. "Vitamin D and calcium supplementation reduces cancer risk: Results of a randomized trial." *American Journal of Clinical Nutrition* 2007;85(6):1586–91.

Lefkowitz ES, Garland CF. "Sunlight, vitamin D, and ovarian cancer mortality rates in US women." *International Journal of Epidemiology* 1994;23:1133–36.

Palmer HG, Larriba MJ, Garcia JM, Ordonez-Moran P, et al. "The transcription factor SNAIL represses vitamin D receptor expression and responsiveness in human colon cancer." *Nature Medicine* 2004;10:917–19.

Peller S, Stephenson CS. "Skin irritation and cancer in the United States Navy." *American Journal of the Medical Sciences* 1937;194:326–33.

Schwartz GG, Whitlatch LW, Chen TC, Lokeshwar BL, Holick MF. "Human prostate cells synthesize 1,25-dihydroxyvitamin D_3 from 25-hydroxyvitamin D_3." *Cancer Epidemiology, Biomarkers and Prevention* 1998;7:391–95.

Spina CS, Tangpricha V, Uskokovic M, Adorinic L, et al. "Vitamin D and cancer." *Anticancer Research* 2006;26(4a):2515–24.

Wactawski-Wende J, Kotchen JM, Anderson GL, et al. "Calcium plus vitamin D supplementation and the risk of colorectal cancer." *New England Journal of Medicine* 2006;354:684–96.

Cardiovascular Health

Bostick R, Kushi LH, Wu Y, Meyer KA, et al. "Relation of calcium, vitamin D and dietary food intake to ischemic heart disease mortality among post menopausal women." *American Journal of Epidemiology* 1999;149:151–61.

Carbone LD, Rosenberg EW, Tolley EA, Holick MF, et al. "25-Hydroxyvitamin D, cholesterol, and ultraviolet irradiation." *Metabolism Clinical and Experimental* 2008; 57:741–48.

Dobnig H, Pilz S, Scharnagl H, Renner W, et al. "Independent association of low serum 25-hydroxyvitamin D and 1,25-dihyroxyvitamin D levels with all-cause and cardiovascular mortality." *Archives of Internal Medicine* 2008; 168(12):1340–49.

Fahrleitner A, Dobnig H, Obernosterer A, et al. "Vitamin D deficiency and secondary hyperparathyroidism are common complications in patients with peripheral arterial disease." *Journal of General Internal Medicine* 2002;17:663–69.

Giovannucci E, Liu Y, Hollis BW, Rimm EB. "25-Hydroxyvitamin D and risk of myocardial infarction in men." *Archives of Internal Medicine* 2008; 168(11):1174–80.

Holick MF. "Sunlight and vitamin D: Both good for cardiovascular health." *Journal of General Internal Medicine* 2002;17(9):733–35.

Jorde R, Bønaa K. "Calcium from dairy products, vitamin D intake, and blood pressure: The Tromsø study." *American Journal of Clinical Nutrition* 2000;71:1530–35.

Krause R, Bühring M, Hopfenmüller W, Holick MF, Sharma AM. "Ultraviolet B and blood pressure." *Lancet* 1998;352(9129):709–10.

Kumar J, Muntner P, Kaskel FJ, Hailpern SM, Melamed ML. "Prevalence and associations of 25-hydroxyvitamin D deficiency in US children: NHANES 2001–2004." *Pediatrics* 2009;124;e362-e370.

Lee JH, O'Keefe JH, Bell D, Hensrud DD, Holick MF. "Vitamin D deficiency: An important, common, and easily treatable cardiovascular risk factor?" *Journal of the American College of Cardiology* 2008 Dec 9;52(24):1949–56.

Lind L, Hanni A, Lithell H, Hvarfner A, et al. "Vitamin D is related to blood pressure and other cardiovascular risk factors in middle-aged men." *American Journal of Hypertension* 1995;8:894–901.

Martins D, Wolf M, Pan D, Zadshir A, et al. "Prevalence of cardiovascular risk factors and the serum levels of 25-hydroxyvitamin D in the United States: Data from the Third National Health and Nutrition Examination Survey." *Archives of Internal Medicine* 2007;167-(11):1159–65.

Melamed ML, Muntner P, Michos ED, Uribarri J, et al. "Serum 25-hydroxyvitamin D levels and the prevalence of peripheral arterial disease: Results from NHANES 2001 to 2004." *Arteriosclerosis, Thrombosis, and Vascular Biology* 2008; 28(6):1179–85.

Pfeifer M, Begerow B, Minne HW, Nachtigall D, Hansen C. "Effects of a short-term vitamin D_3 and calcium supplementation on blood pressure and parathyroid hormone levels in elderly women." *Journal of Clinical Endocrinology and Metabolism* 2001;86:1633–37.

Poole KE, Loveridge N, Barker PJ, Halsall DJ, et al. "Reduced vitamin D in acute stroke." *Stroke* 2006; 37(1):243–45.

Reis JP, von Mühlen D, Miller ER 3rd, Michos ED, Appel LJ. "Vitamin D status and cardiometabolic risk factors in the United States adolescent population." *Pediatrics*. 2009;Aug 3.

Rostand SG. "Ultraviolet light may contribute to geographic and racial blood pressure differences." *Hypertension* 1997;30(2 pt 1):150–56.

Wang TJ, Pencina MJ, Booth SL, Jacques PF, et al. "Vitamin D deficiency and risk of cardiovascular disease." *Circulation* 2008;117(4):503–11.

Zittermann A, Schleithoff SS, Tenderich G, Berthold HK, et al. "Low vitamin D status: A contributing factor in the pathogenesis of congestive heart failure?" *Journal of the American College of Cardiology* 2003;41:105–12.

Immunity

Aloia JR, Li-Ng M. "Epidemic influenza and vitamin D." *Epidemiology and Infection* 2007;12:1–4.

Cannell JJ, Vieth R, Umhau JC, Holick MF, Grant WB, Madronich S, Garland CF, Giovannucci E. "Epidemic influenza and vitamin D." *Epidemiology and Infection* 2006; 134(6):1129–40.

Cantorna MT, Zhu Y, Froicu M, Wittke A. "Vitamin D status, 1,25-dihydroxyvitamin D_3, and the immune system." *American Journal of Clinical Nutrition* 2004;80(suppl):1717S-1720S.

Chan TYK. "Vitamin D deficiency and susceptibility to tuberculosis." *Calcified Tissue International* 2000;66 (6):476–78.

Ginde AA, Mansbach JM, Camargo CA Jr. "Association between serum 25-hydroxyvitamin D level and upper respiratory tract infection in the Third National Health and Nutrition Examination Survey." *Archives of Internal Medicine* 2009 Feb 23;169(4):384–90.

Krause R, Kuhn G, Pose M, Dobberke, et al. "Suberythemal UV-irradiation increases immunological capacity in children with frequent colds." In *Biologic effects of light* 1998. Proceedings of a symposium Basel, Switzerland November 1–3, 1998. M. F. Holick and E. G. Jung, editors. Boston: Kluwer Academic Publishers, 1999:49–51.

Liu PT, Stenger S, Li H, Wenzel L, et al. "Toll-like receptor triggering of a vitamin D–mediated human antimicrobial response." *Science* 2006;311:1770–73.

Kidney Disease

Dusso AS, Brown AJ, Slatopolsky. "Vitamin D." *American Journal of Physiology—Renal Physiology* 2005;289:F8-F28.

Jones G. "Expanding role for vitamin D in chronic kidney disease: Importance of blood 25-OH-D levels and extra-renal 1α-hydroxylase in the classical and nonclassical actions of 1α,25-dihydroxyvitamin D_3." *Seminars in Dialysis* 2007;20(4):316–24.

Muscle Strength

Bischoff-Ferrari HA, Dietrich T, Orav EJ, Hu FB, Zhang Y, Karlson EW, Dawson-Hughes B. "Higher 25-hydroxyvitamin D concentrations are associated with better lower-extremity function in both active and inactive persons aged ≥60 y." *American Journal of Clinical Nutrition* 2004;80(3): 752–58.

Bischoff-Ferrari HA, Dawson-Hughes B, Willett WC, et al. "Effect of vitamin D on falls: A meta-analysis." *Journal of the American Medical Association* 2004;291:1999–2006.

Bischoff-Ferrari HA, Orav EJ, Dawson-Hughes B. "Effects of cholecalciferol plus calcium on falling in ambulatory older men and women." *Archives of Internal Medicine* 2006;166:424–30.

Boland R. "Role of vitamin D in skeletal muscle function." *Endocrine Reviews* 1986;7:434–38.

Broe KE, Chen TC, Weinberg J, Bischoff-Ferrari HA, et al. "A higher dose of vitamin D reduces the risk of falls in nursing home residents: A randomized, multiple-dose study." *Journal of the American Geriatrics Society* 2007;55(2):234–39.

Holick MF. "Sunlight 'D'ilemma: Risk of skin cancer or bone disease and muscle weakness." *Lancet* 2001;357(9249):4–6.

Pfeifer M, Begerow B, Minne HW, et al. "Vitamin D status, trunk muscle strength, body sway, falls, and fractures among 237 postmenopausal women with osteoporosis." *Experimental and Clinical Endocrinology and Diabetes* 2001;109:87–92.

Pfeifer M, Begerow B, Minne H, Abrams C, et al. "Effects of a short-term vitamin D and calcium supplementation on body sway and secondary hyperparathyroidism in elderly women." *Journal of Bone and Mineral Research* 2000;15:1113–15.

Visser M, Deeg DJ, Lips P, Longitudinal Aging Study Amsterdam. "Low vitamin D and high parathyroid hormone levels as determinants of loss of muscle strength and muscle mass (sarcopenia): Longitudinal Aging Study Amsterdam." *Journal of Clinical Endocrinology and Metabolism* 2003;88:5766–72.

Obesity and Metabolic Syndrome

Arunabh S, Pollack S, Yeh J, Aloia JF. "Body fat content and 25-hydroxyvitamin D levels in healthy women." *Journal of Clinical Endocrinology and Metabolism* 2003;88:157–61.

Bell NH, Epstein S, Greene A, Shary J, Oexmann MJ, Shaw S. "Evidence for alteration of the vitamin D-endocrine system in obese subjects." *Journal of Clinical Investigation* 1985;76:370–73.

Ford ES, Ajani UA, McGurie LC, Liu S: "Concentrations of serum vitamin D and the metabolic syndrome among U.S. adults." *Diabetes Care* 2005; 28:1228–30.

Wortsman J, Matsuoka LY, Chen TC, Lu Z, Holick MF. "Decreased bioavailability of vitamin D in obesity." *American Journal of Clinical Nutrition* 2000;72:690–93.

Wortsman J, Matsuoka LY, Chen TC, Zhiren L, Holick MF. "Decreased bioavailability of vitamin D in obesity." *American Journal of Clinical Nutrition* 2000;72:690–93. Erratum in: *American Journal of Clinical Nutrition* 2003;77:1342.

Oral Health

Dietrich T, Nunn M. Dawson-Hughes B, Bischoff-Ferrari HA. "Association between serum concentrations of 25-hydroxyvitamin D and gingival inflammation." *American Journal of Clinical Nutrition* 2005;82: 575–80.

Dietrich T, Joshipura KJ, Dawson-Hughes B, Bischoff-Ferrari IIA. "Association between serum concentrations of 25-hydroxyvitamin D_3 and periodontal disease in the US population." *American Journal of Clinical Nutrition* 2004;80:108–13.

Krall EA, Wehler C, Garcia RI, Harris SS, Dawson-Hughes B. "Calcium and vitamin D supplements reduce tooth loss in the elderly." *American Journal of Medicine* 2001;111:452–56.

Osteomalacia and Fibromyalgia

Glerup H, Mikkelsen K, Poulsen L, Hass E, et al. "Hypovitaminosis D myopathy without biochemical signs of osteomalacic bone involvement." *Calcified Tissue International* 2000 Jun;66(6):419–24.

Plotnikoff GA, and Quigley JM. "Prevalence of severe hypovitaminosis D in patients with persistent, nonspecific musculoskeletal pain." *Mayo Clinic Proceedings* 2003;78:1463–70.

Malabanan AO, Turner AK, Holick MF. "Severe generalized bone pain and osteoporosis in a premenopausal black female: Effect of vitamin D replacement." *Journal of Clinical Densitometry* 1998(1): 201–4.

Holick MF. "Vitamin D deficiency: What a pain it is." *Mayo Clinic Proceedings* 2003;78(12):1457–59.

Osteoporosis, Bone Density, and Calcium Absorption

Abrams SA, Griffin IJ, Hawthorne KM, Gunn SK, et al. "Relationships among Vitamin D levels, parathyroid hormone, and calcium absorption in young adolescents." *Journal of Endocrinology and Metabolism* 2005; 90(10):5576–81.

Araujo AB, Travison TG, Esche GR, Holick MF, et al. "Serum 25-hydroxy-vitamin D and bone mineral density among Hispanic men." *Osteoporosis International* 2009 Feb;20(2):245–55.

Aris RM, Merkel PA, Bachrach LK, Borowitz DS, et al. "Consensus statement: Guide to bone health and disease in cystic fibrosis." *Journal of Clinical Endocrinology and Metabolism* 2005;90(3):1888–96.

Bakhtiyarova S, Lesnyak O, Kyznesova N, Blankenstein MA, Lips P. "Vitamin D status among patients with hip fracture and elderly control subjects in Yekaterinburg, Russia." *Osteoporosis International* 2006;17(3): 441–46.

Beard MK, Lips P, Holick MF, et al. "Vitamin D inadequacy is prevalent among postmenopausal osteoporotic women." *Climateric* 2005;8(Suppl 2):199–200.

Bischoff-Ferrari HA, Willet WC, Wong JB, Giovannucci E, et al. "Fracture prevention with vitamin D supplementation: A meta-analysis of randomized controlled trials." *Journal of the American Medical Association* 2005;293:2257–64.

Bischoff-Ferrari HA, Giovannucci E, Willett WC, Dietrich T, and Dawson-Hughes B. "Estimation of optimal serum concentrations of 25-hydroxyvitamin D for multiple health outcomes." *American Journal of Clinical Nutrition* 2006;84:18–28.

Bischoff-Ferrari HA, Dietrich T, Orav J, Dawson-Hughes B. "Positive association between 25-hydroxyvitamin D levels and bone mineral density: A population-based study of younger and older adults." *Journal of the American Medical Association* 2004;116:634–39.

Chapuy MC, Arlot ME, Duboeuf F, Brun J, et al. "Vitamin D_3 and calcium to prevent hip fractures in elderly women." *New England Journal of Medicine* 1992;327(23):1637–42.

Cooper C, Javaid K, Westlake S, Harvey N, Dennison E. "Developmental origins of osteoporotic fracture: The role of maternal vitamin D insufficiency." *Journal of Nutrition* 2005;135:2728S-2734S.

Dawson-Hughes B, Harris SS, Krall EA, Dallal GE. "Effect of calcium and vitamin D supplementation on bone density in men and women 65 years of age or older." *New England Journal of Medicine.* 1997;337:670–76.

Di Daniele N, Carbonelli MG, Candeloro N, Iacopino L, et al. "Effect of supplementation of calcium and vitamin D on bone mineral density and bone mineral content in peri- and post-menopause women; a double-blind, randomized, controlled trial." *Pharmacological Research* 2004;50:637–41.

Feskanich D, Willett WC, Colditz GA. "Calcium, vitamin D, milk consumption, and hip fractures: A prospective study among postmenopausal women." *American Journal of Clinical Nutrition* 2003;77:504–11.

Glowacki J, Hurwitz S, Thornhill TS, Kelly M, LeBoff MS. "Osteoporosis and vitamin D deficiency among postmenopausal women with osteoarthritis undergoing total hip arthroplasty." *Journal of Bone and Joint Surgery* 2003;85A:2371–77.

Heaney RP, Dowell MS, Hale CA, Bendich A. "Calcium absorption varies within the reference range for serum 25-hydroxyvitamin D." *Journal of the American College of Nutrition* 2003; 22(2), 142–46.

Heaney RP, Davies KM, Chen TC, Holick MF, Barger-Lux MJ. "Human serum 25-hydroxycholecalciferol response to extended oral dosing with cholecalciferol." *American Journal of Clinical Nutrition* 2003;77:204–10.

Terris S. "Calcium plus vitamin D and the risk of fractures." *New England Journal of Medicine* 2006;354(21):2285.

Pregnancy and Lactation

Bodnar LM, Catov JM, Simhan HN, Holick MF, et al. "Maternal vitamin D deficiency increases the risk of preeclampsia." *Journal of Clinical Endocrinology and Metabolism* 2007;92(9):3517–22.

Bodnar LM, Krohn MA, Simhan HN. "Maternal vitamin D deficiency is associated with bacterial vaginosis in the first trimester of pregnancy." *Journal of Nutrition* 2009 Jun;139(6):1157–61.

Camargo Jr CA, Rifas-Shiman SL, Litonjua AA, Rich-Edwards JW, et al. "Prospective study of maternal intake of vitamin D during pregnancy and risk of wheezing illnesses in children at age 2 years." *Journal of Allergy and Clinical Immunology* 2006;117:721–22.

Camargo Jr CA, Rifas-Shiman SL, Litonjua AA, et al. "Maternal intake of vitamin D during pregnancy and risk of recurrent wheeze in children at 3 y of age." *American Journal of Clinical Nutrition* 2007;85(3)788–95.

Merewood A, Mehta SD, Chen TC, Bauchner H, Holick MF. "Association between vitamin D deficiency and primary caesarean section." *Journal of Clinical Endocrinology and Metabolism* 2009 Mar;94(3):940–45.

Hollis BW, Wagner CL. "Assessment of dietary vitamin D requirements during pregnancy and lactation." *American Journal of Clinical Nutrition* 2004;79:717–26.

Hollis BW, Wagner CL. "Vitamin D requirements during lactation: High-dose maternal supplementation as therapy to prevent hypovitaminosis D for both the mother and the nursing infant." *American Journal of Clinical Nutrition* 2004;80:1752S-1758s.

Lee JM, Smith JR, Philipp BL, Chen TC, et al. "Vitamin D deficiency in a healthy group of mothers and newborn infants." *Clinical Pediatrics* 2007; 46:42–44.

McGrath J. "Does 'imprinting' with low prenatal vitamin D contribute to the risk of various adult disorders?" *Medical Hypothesis* 2001;56:367–71.

Pawley N, Bishop NJ. "Prenatal and infant predictors of bone health: The influence of vitamin D." *American Journal of Clinical Nutrition* 2004; 80(suppl):1748S-1751S.

Premenstrual Syndrome

Anderson DJ, Legg NJ, Ridout DA. "Preliminary trial of photic stimulation for premenstrual syndrome." *Journal of Obstetrics and Gynecology* 1997;17(1):76–79.

Lam RW, et al. "A controlled study of light therapy in women with late luteal phase dysphoric disorder." *Psychiatry Research* 1999;86(3):185–92.

Parry BL, et al. "Blunted phase-shift responses to morning bright light in premenstrual dysphoric disorder." *Journal of Biological Rhythms* 1997;12(5): 443–56.

Thys-Jacobs S. "Micronutrients and the premenstrual syndrome: The case for calcium." *Journal of the American College of Nutrition* 2000 Apr;19(2):220–27.

Psoriasis

Bourke JF, Berth-Jones J, Iqbal SJ, Hutchinson PE. "High-dose topical calcipotriol in the treatment of extensive psoriasis vulgaris." *British Journal of Dermatology* 1993;129:74–76.

Holick MF. "Clinical efficacy of 1,25-dihydroxyvitamin D_3 and its analogues in the treatment of psoriasis." *Retinoids* 1998;14:7–12.

Nickoloff B, Schroder J, von den Driesch P, Raychaudhuri S, et al. "Is psoriasis a T-cell disease?" *Experimental Dermatology* 2000;9:359–75.

Perez A, Chen TC, Turner A, Raab R, et al. "Efficacy and safety of topical calcitriol (1,25-dihydroxyvitamin D_3) for the treatment of psoriasis." *British Journal of Dermatology* 1996;134:238–46.

Perez A, Raab R, Chen TC, Turner A, Holick MF. "Safety and efficacy of oral calcitriol (1,25-dihydroxyvitamin D_3) for the treatment of psoriasis." *British Journal of Dermatology* 1996;134:1070–78.

Rickets

DeLucia MC, Mitnick ME, Carpenter TO. 2003. "Nutritional rickets with normal circulating 25-hydroxyvitamin D: A call for reexamining the role of dietary calcium intake in North American infants." *Journal of Clinical Endocrinology and Metabolism* 2003;88:3539–45.

Hess AF, Unger LJ. "The cure of infantile rickets by sunlight." *Journal of the American Medical Association* 1921;77:39–41.

Hess AF, Unger LJ. "Use of the carbon arc light in the prevention and cure of rickets." *Journal of the American Medical Association 1922*; 78:1596–98.

Holick MF. "Resurrection of vitamin D deficiency and rickets." *Journal of Clinical Investigation* 2006;116(8):2062–72.

Holick MF, Lim R, Dighe AS. "Case 3–2009: A 9-month-old boy with seizures." *New England Journal of Medicine* 2009;360:398–407.

Huldschinsky K. "Heilung von Rachitis durch Kunstliche Hohensonne." *Deutsche Med Wochenschr* 1919; 45:712–13.

Huldschinsky, K. "The ultra-violet light treatment of rickets." New Jersey: Alpine Press, 1928, 3–19.

Kreiter SR, Schwartz RP, Kirkman HN, Charlton PA, et al. "Nutritional rickets in African American breast-fed infants." *Journal of Pediatrics* 2000;137:2–6.

Pettifor JM. "Vitamin D deficiency and nutritional rickets in children in vitamin D." In *Vitamin D*, second edition. David Feldman, J. Wesley Pike, Francis H. Glorieux, eds. Boston: Elsevier Academic Press, 2005, 1065–84.

Sniadecki J. Jerdrzej Sniadecki (1768–1838) on the cure of rickets. (1840) Cited by W. Mozolowski. *Nature* 1939; 143:121–24.

Wagner CL, Greer FR; American Academy of Pediatrics Section on Breastfeeding; American Academy of Pediatrics Committee on Nutrition. "Prevention of rickets and vitamin D deficiency in infants, children, and adolescents." *Pediatrics* 2008 Nov;122(5):1142–52.

Skin Cancer

Berwick M, Armstrong BK, Ben-Porat L et al. "Sun exposure and mortality from melanoma." *Journal of the National Cancer Institute* 2005;97, 195–99.

Bikle D. "Vitamin D receptor, UVR, and skin cancer: A potential protective mechanism." *Journal of Investigative Dermatology* 2008;128:2357–61.

Black H, et al. "Evidence that a low-fat diet reduces the occurrence of nonmelanoma skin cancer." *International Journal of Cancer* 1995;62(2):165–69.

Garland FC, Garland CF. "Occupational sunlight exposure and melanoma in the U.S. Navy." *Archives of Environmental Health* 1990;45, 261–67.

Kennedy C, Bajdik CD, Willemze R, de Gruijl FR, Bavinck JN. "The influence of painful sunburns and lifetime of sun exposure on the risk of actinic keratoses, seborrheic warts, melanocytic nevi, atypical nevi and skin cancer." *Journal of Investigative Dermatology* 2003;120(6):1087–93.

Newton-Bishop JA, Beswick S, Randerson-Moor J, Chang YM, et al. "Serum 25-hydroxyvitamin D$_3$ levels are associated with breslow thickness at presentation and survival from melanoma." *Journal of Clinical Oncology* 2009 Nov 10;27(32):5439–44.

Ziegler A, Jonason AS, Leffell DJ, Simon JA, et al. "Sunburn and p53 in the onset of skin cancer." *Nature* 1994;372:773–76.

Tanning Bed Therapy

Koutkia P, Lu Z, Chen TC, Holick MF. "Treatment of vitamin D deficiency due to Crohn's disease with tanning bed ultraviolet B radiation." *Gastroenterology* 2001;121:1485–88.

Tangpricha V, Turner A, Spina C, Decastro S, et al. "Tanning is associated with optimal vitamin D status (serum 25-hydroxyvitamin D concentration) and higher bone mineral density." *American Journal of Clinical Nutrition.* 2004;80:1645–49.

Peterson CA, Heffernan MF, Sisk KA, and Ring SM. "The effects of regular tanning bed use and increased vitamin D status on serum markers of bone turnover in healthy adult women." *Clinical Medicine: Women's Health* 2009:2 1–7.

Type-2 Diabetes

Borissova AM, Tankova T, Kirilov G, Dakovska L, Kovachevas R. "The effect of vitamin D$_3$ on insulin secretion and peripheral insulin sensitivity in type 2 diabetic patients." *International Journal of Clinical Practice* 2003;57:258–61.

Boucher BJ. "Inadequate vitamin D status: Does it contribute to the disorders comprising syndrome X?" *British Journal of Nutrition* 1998;80:585.

Chiu KC, Chu A, Go VLW, Saad MF. "Hypovitaminosis D is associated with insulin resistance and β cell dysfunction." *American Journal of Clinical Nutrition* 2004;79:820–25.

Isai G, Giorgino R, and Adami S. "High prevalence of hypovitaminosis D in female type 2 diabetic population." *Diabetes Care* 2001;24:1496–98.

Kumar S, Davies M, Zakaria Y, et al. "Improvement in glucose tolerance and beta-cell function in a patient with vitamin D deficiency during treatment with vitamin D." *Postgraduate Medical Journal* 1994;70:440–43.

Oh J, Weng S, Felton SK, Bhandare S, et al. "1,25(OH)2 vitamin D inhibits foam cell formation and suppresses macrophage cholesterol uptake in patients with type 2 diabetes mellitus." *Circulation* 2009 Aug 25;120(8): 687–98.

Pittas AG, Dawson-Hughes B, Li T, Van Dam RM, Willett WC, et al. "Vitamin D and calcium intake in relation to type 2 diabetes in women." *Diabetes Care* 2006;29(3):650–56.

Pittas AG, Lau J, Hu FB, Dawson-Hughes B. Review: The role of vitamin D and calcium in type 2 diabetes. A systematic review and meta-analysis." *Journal of Clinical Endocrinology and Metabolism* 2007;92:2017–29.

Schwalfenberg G. "Vitamin D and diabetes: Improvement of glycemic control with vitamin D_3 repletion." *Canadian Family Physician* 2008;54:864–66.

Scragg R, Holdaway I, Singh V, et al. "Serum 25-hydroxyvitamin D_3 levels decreased in impaired glucose tolerance and diabetes mellitus." *Diabetes Research and Clinical Practice* 1995;27:181–88.

Vitamin D_2 vs. D_3

Holick MF, Biancuzzo RM, Chen TC, Klein EK, et al. "Vitamin D_2 is as effective as vitamin D_3 in maintaining circulating concentrations of 25-hydroxyvitamin D." *Journal of Clinical Endocrinology and Metabolism* 2008;93(3):677–81.

Armas LAG, Hollis B, Heaney RP. "Vitamin D2 is much less effective than vitamin D3 in humans." *Journal of Clinical Endocrinology and Metabolism* 2004;89:5387–91.

Vitamin D Deficiency and Intoxication

Bodnar LM, Simhan HN, Powers RW, Frank MP, et al. "High prevalence of vitamin D insufficiency in black and white pregnant women residing in the northern United States and their neonates." *Journal of Nutrition* 2007; 137:447–52.

Calvo MS, Whiting SJ, Barton CN. "Vitamin D intake: A global perspective of current status." *Journal of Nutrition* 2005;135:310–16.

Dawson-Hughes B, Heaney RP, Holick MF, Lips P, et al. "Estimates of optimal vitamin D status." *Osteoporosis International* (Editorial) 2005;16:713–16.

El-Hajj Fuleihan G, Nabulsi M, Choucair M, et al. "Hypovitaminosis D in healthy school children." *Pediatrics* 2001;107:E53.

Ginde AA, Liu MC, Camargo Jr. CA. "Demographic differences and trends of vitamin D insufficiency in the US population, 1988–2004." *Archives of Internal Medicine* 2009 Mar 23;169(6):626–32.

Gordon CM, DePeter KC, Estherann G, Emans SJ. "Prevalence of vitamin D deficiency among healthy adolescents." *Archives of Pediatrics and Adolescent Medicine* 2004;158: 531–37.

Gordon CM, Feldman HA, Sinclair L, Williams AL, et al. "Prevalence of vitamin D deficiency among healthy infants and toddlers." *Archives of Pediatrics and Adolescent Medicine* 2008;162(6):505–12.

Grant WE, Garland CF and Holick MF. "Comparisons of estimated economic burdens due to insufficient solar ultraviolet irradiance and vitamin D and excess solar UV irradiance for the Untied States." *Photochemistry and Photobiology* 2005;81(6):1276–86.

Hanley DA, Davison KS. "Vitamin D insufficiency in North America." *Journal of Nutrition* 2005;135:332–37.

Harris SS, Dawson-Hughes B. "Seasonal changes in plasma 25-hydroxyvitamin D concentrations young American black and white women." *American Journal of Clinical Nutrition* 1998;67(6):1232–36.

Holick MF. "Too little vitamin D in premenopausal women: Why should we care?" *American Journal of Clinical Nutrition* 2002;76:3–4.

Holick MF, Jenkins M. *The UV Advantage*. New York: iBooks; 2003.

Holick MF. "Sunlight and vitamin D for bone health and prevention of autoimmune diseases, cancers, and cardiovascular disease." *American Journal of Clinical Nutrition* 2004;80:1678S-1688S.

Holick MF, Siris ES, Binkley N, Beard MK, et al. "Prevalence of vitamin D inadequacy among postmenopausal North American women receiving osteoporosis therapy." *Journal of Clinical Endocrinology and Metabolism* 2005;90:3215–24.

Holick MF. "High prevalence of vitamin D inadequacy and implications for health." *Mayo Clinic Proceedings* 2006;81(3):353–73.

Holick MF. "Vitamin D deficiency." *New England Journal of Medicine* 2007;357:266–81.

Holick MF, Chen TC. "Vitamin D deficiency: A worldwide problem with health consequences." *American Journal of Clinical Nutrition* 2008; 87(4):1080S-6S.

Jacobus CH, Holick MF, Shao Q, Chen TC, et al. "Hypervitaminosis D associated with drinking milk." *New England Journal of Medicine* 1992; 326:1173–77.

Koutkia P, Chen TC, Holick MF. "Vitamin D intoxication associated with an over-the-counter supplement." *New England Journal of Medicine* 2001;345(1):66–67.

Malabanan A, Veronikis IE, Holick MF. "Redefining vitamin D insufficiency." *Lancet* 1998;351:805–6.

Mansbach JM, Ginde AA, and Carmargo Jr. CA. "Serum 25-hydroxyvitamin D levels among US children aged 1 to 11 Years: Do children need more vitamin D?" *Pediatrics* Nov. 2009;124:1404–10.

Park S, Johnson MA. "Living in low-latitude regions in the United States does not prevent poor vitamin D status." *Nutrition Reviews* 2005;63:203–9.

Sullivan SS, Rosen CJ, Halteman WA, Chen TC, Holick MF. "Adolescent girls in Maine at risk for vitamin D insufficiency." *Journal of the American Dietetic Association* 2005;105:971–74.

Tangpricha V, Pearce EN, Chen TC, Holick MF. "Vitamin D insufficiency among free-living healthy young adults." *American Journal of Medicine* 2002;112(8):659–62.

Vitamin D Nutrition

Chandra P, Wolfenden LL, Ziegler TR, Tian J, et al. "Treatment of vitamin D deficiency with UV light in patients with malabsorption syndromes: A case series." *Photodermatology, Photoimmunology, and Photomedicine* 2007; 23(5):179–85.

Chen TC, Chimeh F, Lu Z, Mathiew J, et al. "Factors that influence the cutaneous synthesis and dietary sources of vitamin D." *Archives of Biochemistry and Biophysics* 2007;460(2):213–17.

Holick MF, Shao Q, Liu WW, Chen TC. "The vitamin D content of fortified milk and infant formula." *New England Journal of Medicine* 1992;326:1178–81.

Tangpricha V, Koutkia P, Rieke SM, Chen TC, et al. "Fortification of orange juice with vitamin D: A novel approach to enhance vitamin D nutritional health." *American Journal of Clinical Nutrition* 2003;77:1478–83.

Vieth R, Garland C, Heaney R, et al. "The urgent need to reconsider recommendations for vitamin D nutrition intake." *American Journal of Clinical Nutrition* 2007;85:649–50.

Vitamin D Skin Synthesis

Clemens TL, Henderson SL, Adams JS, Holick MF. "Increased skin pigment reduces the capacity of skin to synthesis vitamin D_3." *Lancet* 1982;1(8263): 74–76.

Holick MF, MacLaughlin JA, Clark MB, Holick SA, et al. "Photosynthesis of previtamin D_3 in human skin and the physiologic consequences." *Science* 1980;210:203–5.

MacLaughlin J, Holick MF. "Aging decreases the capacity of human skin to produce vitamin D_3." *Journal of Clinical Investigation* 1985;76:1536–38.

Matsuoka LY, Ide L, Wortsman J, MacLaughlin J, Holick MF. "Sunscreens suppress cutaneous vitamin D₃ synthesis." *Journal of Clinical Endocrinology and Metabolism* 1987;64:1165–68.

Webb AR, Kline L, Holick MF. "Influence of season and latitude on the cutaneous synthesis of vitamin D_3: Exposure to winter sunlight in Boston and Edmonton will not promote vitamin D_3 synthesis in human skin." *Journal of Clinical Endocrinology and Metabolism* 1988;67:373–78.

INDEX